Understanding the Autopsy

UNDERSTANDING THE AUTOPSY

Samuel B. Burgess, M.D.

Celo Valley Books
Burnsville, North Carolina

Copies of this book may be purchased by sending $22.50 to the author at: Dr. Samuel B. Burgess, 108 Medford Leas, Medford NJ 08055.

Printed with soy ink on recycled paper.

ISBN 0-923687-26-2
Library of Congress Catalog Card Number 92-74142

Printed in the United States of America

TO JANE

There once was a professor who dedicated his book, "To my wife, without whose constant interruptions, this book would have been finished in half the time." In this case, quite the opposite is true; without my wife's encouragement, enthusiasm, and constant helpfulness, this book probably would not have been written.

TABLE OF CONTENTS

PREFACE

The question of granting autopsy permission upon the death of a family member is a problem which may face anyone, often suddenly, and often people are ill-prepared to respond. Many do not understand what is done in an autopsy, or why the investigation is so important to family members, and to society generally.

This book undertakes to develop an understanding of autopsy, and its related factors. It is directed to a readership of intellectually active people who wish to learn about this important procedure, and particularly to those professionals who must advise people — clergy, lawyers, and social workers — and others who need to be informed on this subject. Even doctors, nurses, and hospital administrators are often not as knowledgeable as they should be.

The public interest needs autopsies in a number of ways. Springing to mind is the medical-legal (forensic) investigation of homicide which features so largely in detective fiction, and which is so important in real life. Other aspects are even more important, such as the identification of infectious disease, and hazards of toxic substances. Most important from a public viewpoint is the function of the autopsy in medical education and research. It has been truly said that autopsy is responsible for fully ninety percent of the medical advances made through the years, and the need continues, in spite of CAT scans and NMR studies. Medical education is greatly handicapped if autopsies are not done. Lastly, the autopsy serves as nothing else can, as a device for assessing the quality of medical care.

On a personal basis, the autopsy is part of the heritage of the family. Studies have shown that many autopsies have unexpected findings and significant differences from the diagnoses made before death. The family deserves to understand the cause of death, and needs to know of any hereditary or familial disease. Often, significant abnormalities are discovered by autopsy, sometimes not of direct importance in the death, but of great importance to others with the same heredity.

The attitude of some doctors that "we know why he died; there's no need for autopsy" is reprehensible. No doctor knows anything that unequivocally; and regrettably, some doctors seem afraid that the autopsy may reveal that they haven't been as smart as they would like people to think. The doctor who discourages an autopsy may have something to conceal.

Finally, the development of new medications and treatments make autopsies even more important. Every medication or surgical operation has some effect on the anatomy or physiology, and only by autopsy can these be fully understood. By putting together the findings from a series of autopsies, physicians may find unsuspected effects of medications or surgical procedures; the collection, storage, and retrieval of information from many autopsies is of greatest importance.

The person who reads this book in hopes of titillation or the thrill of blood and gore is in for a disappointment. There is nothing here that will shock or disgust. But the person who takes up this book in the hope of learning something about the important social function of the autopsy may achieve some satisfaction.

Samuel B. Burgess, M.D.
Medford, New Jersey, U.S.A.
January 1993

CHAPTER ONE

INTRODUCTION

This book is propaganda. I think that the reader should be warned at the start that I am writing from a definite bias in favor of the performance of autopsies. I believe that my reasons are sound and my conclusions fully justified, and I am convinced that the performance of autopsies is an important procedure; important in the advance of medical knowledge and in the health care of people generally.

The number of autopsies done has never been sufficient for the optimum development of an understanding of disease. It approached a satisfactory number in the period just after World War II in the United States, and in a few other countries, but even then, in most parts of the world the number of autopsies was far below the number needed. Recently, even in the United States, there has been a decline in the number of autopsies for a variety of reasons (which I will discuss), and I am hoping that this book, in its small way, will help to reverse the trend. Since I am retired, I cannot be accused of seeking to profit from an increase in business; indeed, because I always worked on a salaried basis, I rarely received any remuneration from autopsies except for the medical-legal cases I performed for the local government. No, my purpose in this book is to help people understand the what and the why of autopsy procedures in hopes that more autopsies will be done, and that medical knowledge will thereby be increased.

What is autopsy? Autopsy is the examination of a dead body, by external examination and by dissection of the organs, in order to determine the cause of death, to observe the changes brought about by disease, and to confirm or deny the conclusions made by the doctor who treated the patient in life as to his impression of the cause of death. Sometimes, autopsy is performed to document a crime for the legal authorities, to assist in the collection of insurance, or to protect the public in cases of suspected contagious disease. But most autopsies are performed on hospital deaths for the purpose of furthering medical knowledge.

I am no Greek scholar — there are few around today — but I understand that the word autopsy comes from the Greek word *autopsia;* this is made up *auto-,* which means self, and *-opsia,* which means seeing. Therefore the word means "to see for oneself". When the pathologist does a postmortem examination, he is seeing for himself what conditions, especially internal conditions, produced the signs and symptoms which were described by the clinician from taking the patient's history and by the physical examination: listening with his stethoscope (auscultation), thumping the patient's chest (percussion), feeling as deeply as possible into the patient's abdomen (palpation) and many other maneuvers. The doctor who makes a diagnosis by such examination is inferring from previous experience, rather than actually seeing. The pathologist at the autopsy table who removes and dissects is observing; he sees with his own eyes.

Of course, *autopsy* may be applied to examinations other than the examination of a body after death; the scene of a murder or a fire may be said to be autopsied. But this book will deal only with the postmortem examination of dead bodies.

Any chapter labeled *Introduction* should be just that; it should introduce the subject to be discussed, and it should introduce the author, and reveal the background from which he is writing. It should also give a view of what I propose to do in the subsequent chapters. I have already introduced the subject, so perhaps the reader will forgive me if I introduce myself.

I am a physician, specializing in the branch of medicine called pathology. I am a physician, and became so, not only from a real desire to become a physician, but also because my father was a physician. Any profession through which I could feel that

I was really helping mankind might have served as well, but medicine was and is a profession which clearly operates to serve the best interests of mankind, so I followed that common sociological practice of following in my father's footsteps. I could be accused of being starry-eyed about the profession of medicine; I felt when I entered training to become a doctor that I was interested in trying, in my own feeble way, to make the world a better place to live in, and I still feel the same way about medicine today. That is not to say that I don't recognize the venal and unscrupulous motives of a small minority of my profession, whose presence within it leads to cynical and critical remarks about doctors generally. I insist, however, that physicians, with few exceptions, are truly dedicated to the healing of the sick, the comfort of the dying, and the prevention of disease.

As I have said, another profession which led to helping mankind might have been just as satisfying to me as medicine. And there are opportunities to serve through many other occupations. Obviously, the callings of the clergyman, the social worker, the teacher, and many others are a matter of real dedication for most of their practitioners, and opportunities for service are found in practically every field of endeavor. I tried secondary-school teaching myself before medical school, but did not do very well, and I made other career experiments before medical training which were not, probably through my own inadequacy, very successful. I'm glad that the doors to medicine opened to me, because, while I was not so brilliant as to become famous, I was conscientious and useful. I feel satisfied that the world is an ever-so-slightly better place as a consequence of my work. Who can ask for more?

I like to say that I am a physician because my great-grandfather was an artist. It is not unusual to find a doctor here or there in one's genealogical chart, but my own direct involvement may be traced to one Dr. Lucius Manlius Sargent, Jr. of Boston. He was apparently a somewhat undisciplined young man who had some difficulty sticking with his education, which led to a departure from Harvard College without graduating. To quote from a manuscript memoir written by his father: "Commenced his education with Rev. W.A. Stearns of Cambridgeport in October 1836. Ran away from Mr. Stearns, as I did, nearly fifty years before from Rev. Dr. Harris. Recommenced with Mr. Dillaway of Roxbury — dissatisfied and parted. Resumed his studies with Mr. Stephen M. Weld of Roxbury — offended Mr. W. by putting frogs in the desk of Usher Davis. Mr. W. requested me to remove him — persuaded Mr. W. to try him again. Mr. W. subsequently offered him at Harvard College. He was admitted freshman. Withdrawn from the University at the request of the Faculty, for inattention, having remained there about the same time as myself. Took a fancy for the sea, & went, before the mast, to Liverpool, in the ship *Anglo Saxon,* Captain Gordon, & returned a steerage passenger, in another vessel, having a desire to see something of life, in this humble phase. After his return, having a turn & taste for the fine arts, he took lessons of Mr. H. Vantin; & proposes, like his uncle, Henry Sargent, who thought well of his capability in this line, to become a painter."

L.M. Sargent, Jr. became an artist and illustrator, exercising a talent which had appeared in several members of his family, and was to appear once again in my distant cousin, John Singer Sargent. As artists will, my great-grandfather decided to take a course in anatomy, for the purpose of improving his ability to draw the human form, and through the anatomy course, he was drawn into completing the entire course of medical school training; he graduated from Harvard Medical School in class of 1858. Harvard College later awarded him his bachelor's degree on the basis of his good medical school record, as a member of the class of 1848. His medical school notebooks are delightfully illustrated with appropriate medical diagrams and drawings, and with caricatures of some of his professors, such as the famous Dr. Bigelow, and Dr. Oliver Wendell Holmes.

So my great-grandfather practiced medicine in the Boston area for several years, and was appointed as Artist to the Massachusetts General Hospital, making him, as far as I can find out, the first professional medical illustrator in the United States. But the Civil War broke out, and in a burst of patriotism, he joined the Medical Department. This service was apparently unsatisfactory, because he was given little to do, and was kept in Boston, so in 1862, he resigned his commission as a surgeon, and was commissioned captain in the Massachusetts Cavalry, under the command of his half brother, General Horace Binney Sargent. He was shot through the chest at Aldie, Virginia in June 1862, "the bullet passing entirely through his body, and being found in his boot;" he recovered and rejoined his unit. He was killed at Bellfield, Virginia on December 9, 1864, having risen to the rank of lieutenant colonel.

The point of this interesting yarn is that my great-grandfather's brief career in medicine led his son George into selecting medicine as a profession, and my father, who had expected to become a forester, changed his choice to medicine, at least in part because of his Uncle George. So I became a doctor because my great-grandfather was an artist. The same influence apparently operated on others, since my brother, my niece, and a cousin are all physicians.

Dr. Sargent's training and medical practice began at just the time that pathology was coming under the tremendous influence of Dr. Rudolf Virchow of Berlin, and among the things that have come down to me from my great-grandfather is a case of autopsy instruments, including one instrument which is now listed in some equipment catalogues as "Virchow's skullbreaker," a chisel with a cross-handle, used to open the bony skull, as I will describe in chapter three. The presence of this instrument in Boston, so soon after its introduction in Berlin, is testimony to the rapidity that medical knowledge was dispersed in the mid-nineteenth century. The instrument case also illustrates that, while there was not an established specialty of pathology in Boston at that time, many physicians were earnest anatomists and proto-pathologists, trying to understand diseases with which they were faced in their practice, and the performance of autopsies was not uncommon at that time.

My great-uncle George was principally a surgeon, but my father, as I will mention in chapter seven, became a pathologist. He trained in Boston, and went to Montreal as Pathologist of the Montreal General Hospital and Assistant Professor of Pathology at McGill Medical School. He found that his eyesight would not keep up with the demands of the microscope, and switched (as one could in those days) to internal medicine. He rose to be an important and influential person in this field, and served on the American Board of Internal Medicine, being one of the few ever to serve on the board who did not hold a medical school professorship; his practice was in Providence, R.I., where there was no medical school. He was an educator par excellence, however, serving as Director of Medical Education in several Providence-area hospitals, and doing extensive work in the reeducation of European physicians who had been displaced during World War II.

I was consequently led to internal medicine, and after medical school, asked my father's advice about appropriate post-doctoral training. He pointed out that most of the really great internists of the past were trained in pathology and that one year of pathology was acceptable for the Board of Internal Medicine, along with two more years of residency in medicine. So to pathology I went, and soon realized that this was my real calling. After a year of rotating internship and four years of pathology residency, I served as pathologist in large chronic-disease hospitals and busy city hospitals. I was Chief of Laboratory Service in a large veterans' hospital, but I found that my true love was the community hospital, so the last twenty years of my practice was working, largely without any physician associates, as Laboratory Director in a sixty-nine-bed general hospital, which grew to 101 beds before I retired. I used to boast that I was the pathologist in the smallest hospital with a full-time pathologist, a position which I delighted in, because I could know just about everything that was happening in the hospital, and feel close to the entire medical staff.

I should say a few words about the medical specialty of pathology. *Pathology* means "the study or knowledge of disease," and the practice of pathology is exactly that. The pathologist occupies himself with the formation of diagnoses through the observations he is able to make in his laboratory. Often he will, on the invitation of the attending physician, examine a living patient at the bedside, and this is important in understanding the problems of day-to-day care of the sick, but most of his work is in the laboratory, examining specimens of tissue removed by the surgeons, studying the characteristics of the blood — the cellular elements and the chemical constituencies — and reviewing other body fluids and solids for all the abnormalities which can help in making a diagnosis.

A diagnosis of disease by the doctor in clinical practice is made on three contrasting bases. First, the determination of the history of the malady through a careful interview with the patient. I remember my medical school professor saying, "Listen to the patient, he is telling you the diagnosis." A carefully done history often makes the diagnosis by itself, and generally excludes a large number of alternative conclusions if it doesn't exactly pinpoint the diagnosis.

The second basis of diagnosis rests upon the physical examination; many astute inferences may be made by feeling, thumping, listening (assisted by a stethoscope), and even smelling; a diagnosis of diabetic coma has often been made quickly and accurately through the odor of acetone which pervades the patient's room. And the diagnosis of alcoholism is often made by nonphysicians through use of the nose.

The third aspect of diagnosis is through the use of special tests. X-ray pictures, radioisotope scans, computer-assisted tomography (CAT scans), and other sophisticated procedures are becoming more and more common, but the laboratory remains the principal contributor to this aspect of diagnosis. Almost without exception, the patient on entering the hospital has blood drawn and urine collected for laboratory study, and often other specimens, such as swabs for bacteriology, syringes of spinal fluid, or small portions of tissue called biopsies, are submitted to the laboratory.

The pathologist is in charge of the laboratory; all items are examined personally by the pathologist or by the technicians who work directly under his supervision. Generally the tissue specimens are examined by the pathologist himself, but he depends on his staff for much of the chemistry, bacteriology, hematology, and so on. The pathologist selects the analysis methods to be used, he should be able to perform all of the tests he asks his technicians to do, and he must review the results of all tests done under his supervision.

The pathologist is the doctor's doctor. His responsibility is to the members of the medical staff of the hospital he serves. Of course, he has a responsibility to patients, both generally and specifically, but he primarily serves the doctor by assisting him to make the diagnosis. He should talk to the patient only with the permission of the attending physician, so it is not surprising that he loses contact with sick patients, and that he is deprived of the satisfaction which some doctors value more highly than fine gold or any other reward, the joy of having the patient say, "Oh, Doctor, aren't you wonderful!"

The pathologist is also the policeman, or at least the detective, of the medical staff. His vantage point is such that he can see if the practice of any member of the medical staff is not up to acceptable standards. He reviews the performance of surgery in the hospital, and reports to the medical staff's tissue committee if Surgeon A is performing inappropriate operations; if Internist B seems to be ordering unjustifiable transfusions, he calls that to the attention of the medical audit committee. The pathologist is indispensable in maintaining high standards of medical practice, and he should always be prepared to protect the public from the incompetent doctor, just as he should protect the doctor from the patient who brings an unjustified malpractice action.

The pathologist must be the servant of truth. There have been extensive discussions among physicians, philosophers, and others concerned with medical ethics on just how far the clinical physician must go in telling the truth to his patient. It is generally understood that he has no obligation — indeed, he is prohibited from revealing truths about his patient — to others; in law, this is a privileged communication, and it is clear that the doctor's ability to serve patients would be severely compromised if the patient could not trust his doctor to keep confidential matters confidential. But just how far the doctor should go in telling the truth to his patient is a real problem. Should the dying patient be told he is dying? There seems to be general agreement that there is no necessity to do so if he doesn't ask, but if the patient does ask, there seems general agreement that he should be told.

The real problem comes when the doctor is convinced that a knowledge of the truth in its clear, unvarnished state will substantially hurt the patient. The ancient Hippocratic concept has always been "First, do no harm." Whatever else the doctor does, his primary obligation is to avoid any activity which might hurt the patient, and if he feels that the truth will indeed harm the patient, he must be very cautious in how he responds to a patient's question. Many authorities on medical ethics agree that there is a difference between lying and deception, and that the latter may be used in good conscience to protect the patient from knowledge which might harm him. Others do not agree, and the debate goes on endlessly in medical-ethics discussions.

The pathologist, however, is in a different position. With him, there must be no deception, either self-deception or deception of others. His professional communication is to other doctors, and he does not ordinarily have a doctor-patient relationship with anyone. But most importantly, he has no one except himself to check on the veracity of his professional answers. The clinician has the pathologist looking over his shoulder in all of his hospital cases, and he knows that the conscientious pathologist may catch him if he does anything dishonest or substandard. The pathologist, with no one to review his work, must, through strength of character, adhere to a strict and uncompromising standard of truth if he is to be effective in his work. There is always a temptation to cover up when an error is made, but the pathologist must be ready to declare, "I was wrong; I made a mistake." He is called to the highest standard of truth in all of his dealings, and the pathologist who does not live up to this standard may damage many lives, and in the process, destroy himself.

The report of the autopsy must therefore come as close as possible to "the truth, the whole truth, and nothing but the truth." It is not for the pathologist to modify his report in consideration of whom it may hurt; that concern should be the responsibility of those to whom the report is made. Thus the pathologist's autopsy report should go to the doctor who attended the deceased and not to the family, unless the doctor requests it.

On the other hand, the autopsy report should not go beyond what is known for sure, from personal observation. I had this problem when a patient died shortly after an operation; a particular anesthetic agent had been used, but, unknown to the surgeon and the anesthesiologist, the patient had had a previous operation in another hospital using the same anesthetic. There is wide suspicion that this particular anesthetic, if used twice in a short period, may cause extensive liver damage. At autopsy, I indeed found very marked liver necrosis, and reported that this was the cause of death. While I was convinced that it was the anesthetic agent which indeed caused the death, all I could say in my report was that the cause was liver necrosis; I could make no statement about the anesthesia, since I did not know, of my own observation, that the anesthesia error might have occurred. This did not stop others from making the connection, however, and a substantial malpractice suit resulted, in which my autopsy report was of prime importance. Of course, I regretted having to report the liver damage; the surgeon, his assistant, and the anesthesiologist were all good friends of mine, and were honest and knowledgeable in their handling of the case. They remain my friends to this day, and they understood fully that I could do nothing else except describe my finding honestly and fully. Indeed, I believe that they would not trust me as a pathologist ever again if I had fudged my report so as to head off the malpractice accusation.

The pathologist is generally deeply involved, and is often the pivotal person in a hospital's education program. And he must serve on administrative committees, and function in the medical staff organization. The pathologist should be, and generally is, a most important person in the hospital administration, and the hospital which doesn't have a full-time pathologist is not a complete hospital. Many small hospitals have circuit-riding pathologists who spend one day per week at each of five similar hospitals; such a situation cannot provide good supervision of the technical staff or prompt diagnosis on the tissue specimens, and the hospital, its medical staff, and the general public are poorly served. The pathologist, I might mention, can make a lot of money by riding circuit, but he is not doing the best job. It would be better if such smaller hospitals would attach themselves to larger teaching institutions, and get their pathology services in that way.

One of the most important functions of the pathologist is the performance of autopsies, and that is what this book is about. I am going to review the actual technique of the autopsy, and the history of the procedure. I will explain autopsies in relation to a number of social functions, such as the legal system, the funeral procedure, religion generally and specifically, and other factors.

In my career, I figure that I must have personally performed at least two thousand autopsies, and directed the work of residents under my supervision in the performance of about a thousand more. There were cases of all kinds: young and old; long hospitalizations and sudden deaths; infant, accident, and murder cases; infectious diseases, heart disease and kidney disease; cancers of the lung, the breast, the brain, the bloodstream, and just about everywhere else. Endocrine diseases, metabolic abnormalities, congenital deformities, and all sorts of other conditions leading to death have appeared on my autopsy table. And here I must make what I feel is one of the most important statements I will make in this book: I have never seen an uninteresting autopsy.

Today, there has been a move to question the need for the routine autopsy of hospital deaths. I can do no better than to quote in response, the dictum of Dr. H. Edward MacMahon, the longtime professor of pathology at Tufts University Medical School: "'There are no routine autopsies; there are only routine pathologists." I can only feel sorry for the pathologist who is not interested in performing autopsies on every death on which he can get legal permission, because he is missing such a great deal. Some pathologists, burdened with the tasks of laboratory administration, the development of new tests, the examination of specimens coming from surgical operations, and the general supervision of their staffs of technical personnel, have taken the attitude that there is no reason to autopsy every hospital death. It takes a great deal of time, and the use of expensive supplies and equipment to perform an autopsy, and usually there is no income to be derived from the procedure, either for the pathologist himself or for the hospital. Hospital autopsies are done generally free-of-charge with the purpose of educating the medical staff, and many pathologists derive their income as a proportion of the bills collected as a result of their laboratory activities (not on salary as I was), so they see the autopsy as wasted time.

In response to this attitude, I can only say that I feel that anyone whose activity is directed mostly by the money to be made is to be pitied. Money-grubbing degrades the profession of pathology. Pathologists should be interested primarily in the intellectual exercise and the knowledge to be gained, knowledge which is necessary for the understanding of disease. The old definition of a profession, as opposed to a job or occupation, was an activity where the principal motivation was that of service, not remuneration, and medicine generally, and pathology specifically, should be a profession under this definition. Perhaps that is why I have been happy, throughout my career, to accept appointments with set salaries, rather than those where my pay would come from the specific tests and procedures done by me or under my direction and responsibility. I could have made at least twice the income I made during my professional career if I had insisted on a fee-for-service type of remuneration, rather than a straight salary. I know of many pathologists with incomes well up in the six-figure range, while my income for doing about the same work was well down in the lower half of five figures for most of my earning years.

I've had a fine time doing pathology. It may seem strange to some when I say that I generally enjoy performing an autopsy. I'm not unmindful of the tragedy of each and every death, but I can't change that, and, as with everyone who feels he can do a good job, I enjoy directing the work of the technical staff under my supervision, and I have enjoyed examining the specimens which come from the operating rooms of the hospital. I have particularly enjoyed the give-and-take discussion with other physicians on the medical staff, and the result of my fixed salary position — that my motives were not suspect when I urged that a particular patient needed a specific and often expensive test, because my income remained the same, whether or not that test was done. I enjoyed performing the autopsies on the bodies of those who, in spite of the earnest efforts of the attending physician, came to the inevitable conclusion of death. It gave me a real consciousness of adding, if only in a tiny fragment, to the structure of knowledge by which the medical profession has been able to increase the length and comfort of life.

I've often been asked if there is such a thing as a pathologist who is made uncomfortable by the contemplation of the body on the autopsy table. I must admit that I react emotionally if the patient is young, and especially if the case is a young woman. Suicide and murder are repulsive to me, and the accidental death of the younger person driving home from the high-school prom seems so stupid. But as for the inevitable release of blood and feces during the autopsy procedure, these are things to which the pathologist ordinarily becomes accustomed. There are times when I would rather be in the fresh air than indoors dissecting a body of drowning victim who had been in the water several days, but such problems are soon forgotten in the search for the exact cause and nature of the death. I would much rather perform an autopsy than dissect an amputated leg, because in the latter case, I know that there is a living patient who will spend the rest of his life without that leg. As for performing the autopsy of a family member or close acquaintance, I have never had any problem, nor would most pathologists. The pathologist learns early in his training, that the object on the autopsy table is a dead body; it is not a person. The pathologist is not hardhearted; he merely is able to separate the body from the person in his mind, a thing that is difficult to do the first time one sees a dead body, but which becomes increasingly easy with repetition of the experience.

As I have said, the decrease in the number of autopsies performed is very disturbing to me, and it is the reason for this book. In my discussion of the function of the pathologist, I may have given the impression that the decrease is due to stupid or lazy pathologists, and while this may be a factor, it is far from the most important cause. Many influences have worked together to produce the effect. For instance, the hospital administrator, mindful as he must be of the cost of the autopsy to the hospital and under pressure from his board of trustees to reduce expenses, may openly or through subterfuge, actively discourage autopsies, by finding objections about the legality of the autopsy permission, or some similar obstacle. The costs of the autopsy are not reimbursed by the third-party payers such as insurance companies or Blue Cross. This administrative obstruction did not take place when the Joint Commission for the Accreditation of Hospitals (now the Joint Commission for the Accreditation of Health Organizations) had a standard in effect for the percentage of hospital deaths that had to be autopsied, because the administrator knew that the hospital could lose its accreditation if the standard was not met; he became an enthusiastic advocate of the procedure, and constantly goaded the medical staff into trying for more autopsy permissions.

The withdrawal of the standard for autopsied cases by the Joint Commission for the Accreditation of Hospitals itself was both the cause and the effect of a deterioration of the autopsy procedure. On one hand, the withdrawal reflected a feeling that everything anatomical had already been seen, and that further autopsies would yield diminishing returns for the money spent. On the other hand, the withdrawal itself caused hospitals and their medical staffs to view the need for autopsies less seriously.

Another influence which has caused some decrease in the number of autopsies performed is the feeling on the part of some physicians that the results of the autopsy might be used as evidence to support a malpractice claim by the family of the deceased. The deliberations of the tissue committee of the medical staff are privileged and cannot be subpoenaed, but the report of the autopsy becomes part of the hospital chart, and can be called by the court. There was an explosion of malpractice suits a few years ago, and even today, malpractice awards are of tremendous size, but the number of actions has decreased recently, and countersuits are discouraging new filings. An instance of this is a recent orthopedic case where suit was brought in spite of many reassurances by other physicians that there was no malpractice. The attorney for the plaintiff never examined the hospital chart or engaged expert witnesses, and offered to settle for only $750. The doctor being sued would not permit his insurance carrier to settle, and the case was tried and dismissed. The doctor then sued the plaintiff's attorney for abuse of process, charging that the suit was entered only to harass him into a settlement, and he won $85,000 in damages from the attorney. The wind is beginning to blow from the other direction in malpractice cases today.

I am very doubtful if an autopsy report would be useful in support of a malpractice action if the attending physician has done a proper job; on the other hand, if there was a real case of malpractice, the performance of an autopsy is greatly needed to protect the public from an incompetent physician. Most autopsies will yield information which should be useful in defending against malpractice claims, and actually protect the doctor against unjustified litigation. The obtaining of autopsy permission is evidence of a sincere desire to give the best care possible, and the request for autopsy permission really shows that the doctor wants to do things right. The failure of the doctor to speak to the family after a death to ask that autopsy be done, can easily be interpreted as an attempt at concealment.

I sincerely believe that autopsy is important from many points of view, and there is no good reason not to do the procedure in every case of death, whether in the hospital or outside. There has been a reduction in the understanding and the performance of the procedure, so I am writing in hopes that a better understanding of autopsies by doctors, clergymen, lawyers, and every segment of human society will lead to a better acceptance, and even a wholehearted advocacy of the socially valuable procedure of autopsy.

CHAPTER TWO

HISTORY OF THE AUTOPSY

To consider the history of the autopsy is to consider the history of medicine itself, since the autopsy has been so completely part-and-parcel of every medical advance throughout history. I can touch only a few of the high spots in a chapter as short as this must be; to treat the subject adequately would require a whole book. The result is that I must leave out hundreds of highly significant names of individuals who have contributed so very greatly to the development of medicine through the use of the autopsy. Certain familiar names, such as Pasteur, Semmelweis, and Jenner, will be found to be entirely absent. Surely the autopsy played significant parts in their work, but they did not specifically contribute to the development of autopsy as a technique of medical investigation.

It is difficult to begin a review of the history of autopsy without mouthing some fatuous banalities that have been stated a thousand times. Statements such as "There is clear evidence of at least some rudimentary knowledge of anatomy in prehistoric civilizations as evidenced by archeology" are easy to make and to support, but are hardly definitive and useful in considering the autopsy today. It has been pointed out that Egyptian knowledge of anatomy must have been extensive, because the dead bodies of so many important people were at least semidissected preparatory to mummification, and the viscera placed in separate jars. But this does not mean that there was any real study of disease; indeed, the evidence is to the contrary.

Disease in many so-called primitive civilizations was, and

still is, perceived to be caused by possession by evil spirits, and it is clear that this was the belief in early Egypt, as elsewhere. Possession by demons as a cause of disease survives today in many cultures. One does not have to leave the modern culture of America to find belief in the evil eye, and many of today's beliefs bear a remarkably close resemblance to the primitive concept that evil (or erroneous) thoughts are responsible for disease.

The first step toward making possible the real study of disease — i.e., seeing diseases as physiological mechanisms and as anatomic alterations to be understood, instead of as the actions of a demon to be feared and hopefully cast out — occurred about 400 B.C. on the island of Kos, in the Aegean Sea near Asia Minor. This was at a famous medical school, the first school of scientific medicine whose shining star was Hippocrates. Not only did Hippocrates and his associates turn common thinking around toward real observation and rational treatment, but they did it by bedside teaching, the method which has been so effective over the years since that time, and which today still represents the best in medical instruction. Regrettably, bedside teaching is somewhat in eclipse today, being somewhat overshadowed by laboratory observation and classroom lecture.

It is apparent that even Hippocrates and his brilliant group rarely did any extensive investigation of human anatomy, however. They were restricted by the religious beliefs of the time, particularly the conviction that the intact body of the deceased must be cremated to avoid having the soul condemned to wandering forever on the banks of the River Styx. But it is equally apparent that some human dissection was carried out, that animal dissection was extensive, and that comparative anatomy (the relation between human and animal anatomy) was beginning to be understood.

Another later student of the medical school of Kos is an even more familiar name: Aristotle, who, among his many other accomplishments, was a physician and the primary teacher of young Alexander, who was soon to become the conqueror of most of the known (i.e., Western) world of that day. Alexander's conquests included Egypt, and the Greek advances in medical knowledge were carried there and flourished under the 400-year dynasty founded by Alexander's general, Ptolemy. Investigative human dissection began to be carried out in this period, and great advances made, only to be lost in the destruction of the great library of Alexandria by the Romans in 30 B.C. Indeed, the little that is known about Alexandrian medicine is from Aulus Cornelius Celsus, whose writing mentions the works of seventy-two medical authors, one of whom was Hippocrates, but all the others are known only from Celsus's report.

Claudius Galenus (now universally called simply Galen), born in 130 A.D., made very extensive contributions to the medical knowledge of the day, and his persuasive personality, the firmness of his opinions, and his restrictive philosophical ideas dominated medical thinking for the next thousand years; thus, for all his contributions, he substantially interfered with subsequent medical progress for a very long time. Galen studied at Alexandria, and cites references similar to those reported by Celsus. He undoubtedly profited by the medical knowledge which was present and later lost in recorded form by the Roman destruction. It is clear that Galen did, indeed, perform dissections of animals and that he extended his observations to apply to human anatomy, but there is no good evidence that he performed any dissections of human bodies. His impact on medicine was so great that, for many years after his work, the general attitude seemed to be that Galen had so precisely and accurately defined the whole of medical knowledge that no further investigation needed to be done, which substantially slowed the subsequent development of medical knowledge.

The first real breakthrough in the subsequent sterile period seems to have occurred with Taddeo di Alderetto, who is said to have performed dissections frequently for the instruction of his students at the University of Bologna in 1260. There are occasional references to anatomical studies prior to that date, but there are no organized reports or useful material. The Holy Roman Emperor, Frederick II, had authorized human dissection for the purposes of study shortly before this, and following this approval, anatomic dissection became quite common, if somewhat disorganized, but mainly for the demonstration of normal anatomy rather than for the study of disease. Only occasional references are found to the investigation of the causes of death.

Naturally, the understanding of normal anatomy is essential to the understanding of the alterations of the normal, i.e., the anatomical evidence of disease, and the dissections which were carried out, from the thirteenth century onward were of great importance. Today, the study of normal anatomy is still the initial course of instruction in any medical school, although the time devoted to this subject has been progressively diminished by the pressure of the burgeoning body of knowledge in other fields of medicine which the medical student must absorb in a limited length of time.

In spite of the increasing occurrence of dissection of the bodies of deceased humans, it is clear that the primitive revulsion to this procedure had not disappeared. There was a good deal of public opposition, in spite of the apparent reversal on the part of the Roman church — which had previously held that "the church abhors blood," and that surgery could not be performed, whether the patient was living or dead, by any of the clergy. (In those days, practically all the physicians were members of the clergy.) Even well after the clear approval of autopsies by ecclesiastic authorities, it was found necessary to provide a trapdoor in the floor, next to the autopsy table at the University of Padua, so the body being autopsied could be concealed in the event of a raid.

The selection of bodies for dissection in these early days was largely determined, not by disease to be studied, but by the chances of the social situation; bodies used for dissection were largely those of executed criminals. Indeed, the release of the body for dissection was often thought of as a continuing punishment for misdeeds. Sentences such as condemnation to be "drawn and quartered, and the entrails fed to the dogs" imply that society saw the destruction of the already-dead body as further punishment, and there is evidence that the delivery of the body to the anatomist was, in large part, motivated by a similar spirit. It was not until much later that Burke and Hare furnished bodies to anatomists through acts of murder — they suffocated victims after first rendering them drunk. This, so far as I can determine, is the only case of murdering in order to supply bodies for dissection.

The development of the true autopsy, that is, the anatomic dissection specifically for the study of disease-states manifested before death, began slowly. Pliny credits Herophilus as the first investigator to do this, in the Greco-Alexandrian years before the rise of Rome. He is said to have noted many details such as ligamentous tears associated with hip fractures, and alterations by disease in the anatomy of the eye, the nerves, and the brain. In the sixth century A.D., an outbreak of plague at Constantinople was studied, in part by autopsy, according to Morgagni. In 1410, Pope Alexander V died under suspicious circumstances, and an autopsy was carried out by Pietro d'Argelata with equivocal results. One particularly fascinating case of autopsy was performed in 1533: conjoined ("Siamese") twins had been born on the island of Hispañola, and the question arose as to whether baptism was required for one soul or two. After the death of the infant (or infants, as the question was), an autopsy showed that there were two complete sets of internal organs, so it was decided that the priest had been correct when he performed two baptisms. Some writers have pointed out that this is the only autopsy ever performed to determine the state of the soul.

Gradually, over the succeeding two centuries, autopsies became more common. Public opposition, however, was still strong, and clandestine dissection was more the rule than the exception. The reasons for dissection continued to be generally anatomical, but the use of dissection for the training of artists also came into use extensively. Francis Bacon, in 1623, wrote of the advantages of autopsy in the study of disease, and William Harvey, who in 1628 had finally put down Galen's misconceptions on the nature of blood circulation, also stated, "More can be learned from the dissection of the body of one dead from a chronic malady like consumption, than from the bodies of ten animals."

Anatomic pathology really begins, as a real specialty of medicine, with the publication by Giovanni Battista Morgagni of the results of his lifework, in 1761, when he was seventy-nine years old. Morgagni, a native of Forlì, Italy, became professor at the University of Padua at age thirty-three, and continued until his death at age eighty-nine. During this time, he conducted over seven hundred autopsies, with careful notes and correlation of his findings with the clinical histories of the patients. He presented the first descriptions of diseases such as syphilitic aneurysm, tuberculosis of the kidney, and acute hepatic necrosis, and correctly identified pneumonia with lung consolidation. His work was careful, accurate, and very useful to the physicians of the day — and ever since.

The invention of the microscope had far-reaching effects on the understanding of both the anatomic variations and the bacterial infestations which are characteristic of various diseases. The stories about Anton van Leeuwenhoek have been recounted many times — how he manufactured 247 microscopes with 419 lenses which he ground himself, how he first described spermatozoa, striated muscle, and red blood corpuscles, and divided bacteria into cocci, bacilli, and spirilla. But contrary to popular belief, the credit for the first use of the microscope in the study of disease belongs to Athanasius Kircher, a learned Jesuit priest, physician, musician, and mathematician.

The founder of histology (the study of sectioned and stained tissues under the microscope) was Marcello Malpighi, who was professor of anatomy at Bologna, Pisa, and Messina, and was personal physician to Pope Innocent XII. Malpighi's name survives in the Malpighian layer of the skin, and the Malpighian bodies of the spleen and kidney, and his description of the blood capillaries in 1660 completed the concepts of Harvey on the circulation of the blood. Without the invention of the microscope, anatomic pathology could never have progressed with the speed and completeness that it did. A later chapter details the microscope's history and use.

I cannot begin to mention all of the great pathologists who followed Morgagni and Malpighi, such men as Matthew Baillie, personal physician to King George III of England, and Marie-François Xavier Bichat in France, who made tremendous contributions to the understanding of the anatomic evidence of disease. The period from the late seventeenth century through the early nineteenth century was a period of ferment in many disciplines, and anatomic pathology was no exception. But Rudolf Virchow stood above all the other pathologists of the mid-nineteenth century, and founded the concept of cellular pathology. The concept of the cell had been defined only five years before Virchow's graduation from training, by Schleiden and Schwann. In 1847, Virchow founded the journal, the *Archiv für pathologische Anatomie,* which quickly became known as *Virchow's Archiv*, and is still published today. He began his work by declaring that no investigator is infallible in his conclusions, and that all hypotheses must be checked and rechecked before acceptance. This valuable concept had, surprisingly, never been stated before in the context of medical science. If someone of Virchow's character had been around when Galen was alive, perhaps the progress of medical knowledge would have been faster. Prior to Virchow, medicine had proceeded mostly on crystallized knowledge and hunch, and all too often, on the conclusions reached by a single investigator.

Virchow was continuously engaged in professional controversy while, personally, he was a generous and helpful man. Nevertheless, he set a tone of aggressive sarcasm and scorn of mistakes which dominates the teaching methods of many pathology professors today, giving support to the theory that pathologists become pathologists because they hate people in general, and those nearest them in particular. Virchow began his career by virtually destroying some of the concepts of the great and genial pathologist Carl Rokitansky of Vienna, himself the prosector (one who performs anatomical dissections) in more than thirty thousand autopsies, but who developed and published a paper attributing disease to chemical changes within tissues, humors, and other outmoded ideas. It has been reported that, after Virchow's scathing criticism, Rokitansky was unable to bring himself to read his own paper again. But Virchow also praised much of Rokitansky's other work.

Virchow studied in Berlin, and had his first appointments there. His liberal politics and his readiness to antagonize others led to his removal, and for seven years, he worked at Würzburg before he was invited back to Berlin with great honor and placed in charge of the Pathological Institute which had been built specifically for him. He never left politics, however, and served in the Reichstag from 1880 to 1883. He was also an anthropologist and archeologist (he worked with Schliemann at Troy), and was a sanitarian and epidemiologist within the field of medicine. But his greatest contributions were to pathology, and his students dominated pathology for many years. His students' students dominate pathology today.

With Virchow, anatomic pathology took on practically all the aspects of the practice today. The pathology resident is taught to open the chambers of the heart in the way Virchow did, and the autopsy report is written in the same general style as Virchow's. Even the attitudes encountered in many pathology laboratories derive from Virchow's sarcastic and abrasive method of teaching. The debt that pathology owes to Rudolf Virchow is tremendous, and he is rightly appreciated as the father of modern pathology.

Virchow became a legend in his own time, and remains a legend today. Not long ago, a colleague of mine was traveling in Germany and mentioned to the chambermaid at a hotel that he was a pathologist. Her response seventy-five years after his death, was, "*Wie Virchow?* (like Virchow)?"

Perhaps Virchow's most outstanding student was Julius Cohnheim, who, in turn, became a great teacher, and worked at Kiel, Breslau, and Leipzig. At Breslau, one of his students was William Henry Welch, a native of Norfolk, Connecticut, and a recent graduate of the College of Physicians and Surgeons in New York. In 1884, Welch returned from his studies in Germany to become Professor of Pathology at the newly organized Johns Hopkins Medical School in Baltimore. He was one of the four great teachers who made Johns Hopkins the celebrated medical center it was and is today; the others were Kelly in Obstetrics, Halsted in Surgery, and Osler in Medicine. Welch was a rotund bachelor with a neat beard, and he collected a large group of earnest students, who were known, perhaps inevitably, as "Welch Rabbits"; Welch, himself, was universally known as Popsy.

Welch's students, generally with the obligatory year or more of training in Germany or Austria, spread out over America to the various medical schools, and brought the Virchow techniques to the medical training of the United States and Canada. Among the students who brought the pathology message to my area was Dr. Frank Burr Mallory, who became Chief of Pathology at Boston City Hospital, and under whom my father trained. Dr. Mallory's two sons became famous pathologists, and Dr. G. Kenneth Mallory was Director of the Mallory Institute of Pathology at Boston City Hospital and was my professor of pathology when I was a medical student. Another of Welch's students was Dr. Winternitz of Yale who trained Dr. Paul Rosahn, who in turn, was chief of pathology during my residency training. So, in three ways, I can claim to be a great grandson of Popsy Welch, and a great-great-grandson of the great Rudolf Virchow.

The early years of the twentieth century saw splendid development in the practice of pathology, and in the performance of autopsies. The quality of medical school teaching improved, in large part due to the stimulus of the famous 1910 Flexner Report, in which Abraham Flexner reported on his studies of medical schools. As a result of the Flexner Report, a number of inadequate schools were closed; and today, only Class A medical schools exist in this country, although less-than-satisfactory training is available in Mexico and in the Caribbean for U.S. medical students. Standardization of training at a high level resulted in excellent pathology instruction and the development of the autopsy as a primary teaching mechanism in all of the great medical centers. Students still went to European medical centers for advanced instruction, right up to the outbreak of hostilities in 1939; indeed, my older brother studied pathology in Vienna at this time, one of the last American students to do so as part of post-doctoral training.

The period following World War II saw an explosion of training opportunities, fueled both by government support of returning veterans and by increased emphasis on specialty training. The number of pathologists increased tremendously. The Veterans Administration expanded and began to pay a twenty-five percent addition to the salary of anyone who could show the certificate of any recognized American specialty certification board, and this created an economic stimulus toward specialization; indeed, specialists' incomes became standardized throughout all types of medical practice at a higher level, including pathology, which had been relatively poorly paid.

Another factor caused the supply of pathologists to increase: foreign doctors began migrating to the United States in large numbers. First came the genuine refugees and displaced persons, whose opportunities in their native lands had been cut off. Then came wave upon wave of foreign-trained doctors who saw better opportunities, both professional and financial, in the United States. Many of these immigrant physicians had poor command of the English language, and found that private practice in specialties involving direct patient contact was less likely to succeed as compared with the hospital-based specialties such as radiology, anesthesiology, physiatry — and pathology. For these practices, the communication was mainly with other doctors, and more often than not it was in written form, so the foreign accent was not such a problem; so lots of Egyptians, Filipinos, Bolivians, and the like became pathologists.

With the vast increase of the supply of pathologists, the small hospital which had never had adequate pathology services began to acquire part-time, and then full-time pathologists. The result was that autopsies, which previously had been available only on a difficult-to-arrange basis, and often with long delays which embarrassed the hospital, the funeral director, and the family of the deceased, now became readily and promptly available. The number of autopsies performed rose dramatically. Hospitals took pride in autopsy percentages of fifty, seventy, and even ninety percent of the hospital deaths. The quality of the autopsies also improved, because it became less acceptable to perform an incomplete or cause-of-death-only autopsy. The Virchow-style autopsy report, running to eight or more pages became, while not mandatory, at least much more common.

Today, reaction seems to have set in, and the number of autopsies has decreased. I have discussed elsewhere the many factors leading to this decline in autopsy performance: the lowering of standards, the increased involvement with other laboratory procedures, and the lack of remuneration for the work involved, among other influences. Autopsies, which were performed by prideful specialists eager to show off there expertise, are now relegated to first-year residents; and the attending physicians, who once followed their cases to the autopsy room for conclusion, now rarely even attend the procedure.

There are hopeful signs, however. More and more, editorials and articles are appearing in medical journals and even in the public press, pointing out the need for autopsies and calling for increased performance. So the pendulum swings, and we can look forward to a rebirth of interest in the careful investigation of causes of death and disease.

CHAPTER THREE

THE TECHNIQUE OF AUTOPSY

In this chapter, I will present in detail the actual autopsy procedure. If any reader is disturbed by the description, he can readily skip to the next chapter with the assurance that he is not missing any information which is essential to the understanding of the rest of the book. There are those, however, who would like to know exactly what is done in a general autopsy, and for such interested individuals, this chapter is presented. The forensic autopsy is more complicated, and is discussed in chapter nine.

The typical autopsy takes the pathologist between two and five hours in the autopsy room, and from three to six hours at the microscope, completing the report. It begins with the notification of the prosector — whether he be a pathologist or pathologist in training — of the existence of an autopsy permission from the next-of-kin of some patient recently deceased. In the best circumstances, this notification comes directly from the physician who has cared for the patient, because he is able to explain some of the details of the case and any problems that need to be studied in the particular autopsy. All too often, though, the prosector hears of the pending autopsy through a call from the nurse-supervisor, the charge nurse, or even the hospital telephone operator; in such cases, the prosector is in the dark as to what special problems the autopsy is expected to show. Indeed, on more than one occasion, I have first heard of an autopsy permission through a call from the funeral director, who wants to know when the autopsy will be completed!

Even if the attending physician describes the case in full, the prosector's first move is to obtain the clinical chart and examine it, to find if there are any special problems ahead of him. He also views the signed autopsy permission form, because it is his responsibility to satisfy himself that it is indeed a legal permission; pathologists who proceed with an autopsy on the statement that there is a valid permission but without actually seeing it are asking for trouble.

The prosector notifies the diener (the technical assistant who will help him) and sets the time for the autopsy; he arranges that the attending physician and others interested in the case are notified of the time that the procedure is to begin. In some hospitals, this is done over the public address system with some code (supposed to be understood by only the medical staff) such as "Pathology conference at 8:30 P.M." or "Dr. Post, Dr. Mortimer Post." (How transparent can you get?)

GROSS AUTOPSY

After changing to a scrub suit, the prosector dons his apron and rubber gloves, and begins to examine the external appearance of the body, which the diener has placed on the autopsy table. The table is generally made of stainless steel, with no covering, and some tables are equipped with cross-slats so that the body is suspended over a sheet of running water. The diener has laid out the appropriate instruments, and stands by with a sponge in hand to carry out the prosector's orders. The diener's job is to assist the prosector and to keep the area clean; in some institutions, he has been trained to open the head, and may proceed immediately to this task while the prosector works on the thorax and abdomen.

The prosector examines the external appearance of the body. He looks and feels to answer various questions: Is the body jaundiced? Is the skin dry and atrophic? Is there rigor mortis of the jaws, the arms, or the legs? Is there any ulceration of the skin? Is there any evidence of tumor mass, distention, old surgical scars, or traumatic scars? In short, the body is examined in considerable detail for any external abnormality, with measurement of height, estimate of weight, and a comparison of the prosector's opinion on the body's age with the age recorded in the hospital chart. All sorts of variation from the normal are noted, such as gangrene, unusual hair distribution, eye abnormalities, and, of course, in medical-legal cases particularly, the presence of wounds, bruises, and other signs of trauma. Often it is valuable to photograph external lesions before proceeding further with the autopsy, especially in medical-legal cases.

The pathologist often has a microphone suspended above the table so he can dictate his findings as he identifies them, but I always found it more convenient to perform the whole autopsy, recording only weights and measures on a slip of paper; I found I could recall with complete accuracy all of the significant findings, and visualize the entire autopsy for many hours afterward. It was easier and more satisfactory to organize the report into a coherent story while seated at my desk immediately after the autopsy, than to dictate it in bits and pieces during the process of the actual dissection.

With the external examination complete, the pathologist now proceeds with the incision of the body. A Y-shaped incision is made, starting from each shoulder and joining over the lower end of the breastbone, (the xiphoid process), and continuing straight down to the pubis, passing just to the left of the navel. The incision goes through all the layers of tissue down to the ribs, and entirely through the abdominal wall; the tissues over the chest are cut away from the ribs. In females, some pathologists carry the chest incision from one shoulder, down and around the breasts to the other shoulder, so the incision is in a U-shape, with a tail extending down the abdomen, but my embalmer friends say that this only makes a longer incision that is harder to close, and serves no apparent purpose. If the lady were to be buried in a very low-necked dress, it might possibly help, but such clothing is rarely chosen for a funeral.

The prosector explores the abdomen, feeling for all of the organs and searching for abnormalities. He then cuts the ribs up both sides of the chest and removes the anterior part of the thoracic rib cage; he explores the chest with his hands, and opens the pericardial sac which surrounds the heart, to look for abnormalities there. The heart is then removed by cutting across the large arteries and veins, and the lungs are similarly lifted out by cutting across the windpipe attachments. The interior of the chest cavity is examined, and the neck organs are also explored, generally with the removal of the thyroid gland, and sometimes the parathyroid glands, which are very difficult to find, because they are so small. Great care must be taken not to cut the skin of the neck, which is lifted away in the examination of the neck organs, and the arteries of the neck must be carefully preserved so that the embalmer may accomplish his work, as seen in chapter eleven, where the embalming of the body is described.

The abdominal viscera examination may be done in one of two basic ways. The surgical approach is sometimes used. This consists of removing the organs one by one, starting with the small intestine, which is in the way of the other organs, and proceeding from the front of the abdomen to the back. I prefer, however, to remove all of the abdominal organs in one block, by cutting across the rectum and other pelvic attachments, and dissecting upwards behind all of the organs including the kidneys, which lie back against the rear wall of the body cavity. Then I place this block of organs, front downward, on the table and dissect from the back forward, starting with the aorta and kidneys, and examining the small intestine last. I feel that this approach gives me a better idea of the relationships of the organs to each other.

Now that the body is eviscerated, the abdominal and thoracic cavities are rinsed of blood and debris, and careful inspection of the lining of these cavities is made. At this point, if no examination of the head is permitted, the body is sewed up by the diener, ready to be picked up by the undertaker. If head examination is to be done, an incision is made through the scalp, from behind one ear, over the posterior part of the top of the head, to behind the other ear. The scalp is peeled off the bone, forward and back, and the bony skull is cut with an electric saw in two lines, one just about where the hairline would be, and the other across the back of the skull, meeting the first cut near each ear. The bone can then be removed, and the brain cavity explored, with removal of the brain, and careful examination of the interior of the skull.

The bone can then be replaced and the scalp sewed back into place. The incision is covered by hair and no one can tell if the head has been invaded unless he pulls the ear forward to expose the end of the cut.

The pathologist, while the diener is sewing up the body and cleaning it for the undertaker, goes on to examine the organs one by one. The heart is opened in a standard manner, and the valves, muscles, and coronary arteries checked; multiple cuts are made across the heart muscle to look for fibrous changes, or for the softening and discoloration which are characteristic of the heart attack. The lungs are dissected, following down the air passages and blood vessels, and multiple cuts are made across the lungs, looking for the consolidation of pneumonia, abscess, tumor, or other abnormality. The liver is sliced like a loaf of bread, after the external surfaces are examined, and the gallbladder and bile passages are opened and examined. The spleen is likewise bread-loafed, and multiple cuts are made across the pancreas. The adrenals and kidneys are examined, externally and on the cut surfaces. The esophagus, stomach, small intestine, and large intestine are opened for their entire length, looking for ulcer, tumor, or anything out of the ordinary. The appendix is checked. The urinary bladder, and either the uterus and ovaries or the testicles, as the case may be, are opened and carefully examined. The brain is also examined externally and may be placed whole in formalin solution for hardening and dissection later. This process helps with the dissection because the brain is quite soft in the fresh state, and information may be lost by immediate sectioning. Sometimes immediate examination by multiple cuts is necessary in a particular case, and then it is done as carefully as possible. But however it is done, the coverings are examined, the blood vessels are checked, and then the entire brain is cut at half-inch intervals like a loaf of bread.

Of course, the innumerable details and related maneuvers cannot be described in detail here, and it is not our purpose here to give minute directions on "How To Do an Autopsy", but only a rough sketch of the gross autopsy. The procedure has taken two to five hours up to this point, and the work is only beginning. The pathologist, in checking each organ, has taken a portion of tissue and placed it in a jar of formalin solution; this is a solution of formaldehyde gas in water which fixes the tissue. Fixation is a matter of hardening and stopping all the metabolic processes in the tissue so it will represent the state of the tissue unchanged from the time of the autopsy, even years later. From these tissue blocks, the pathologist chooses smaller pieces for the histology technician to make into tissue samples for the microscope.

MICROSCOPIC AUTOPSY

Histology is a science and an art, and the skilled histology technician can make the pathologist's life a great deal easier. Here is what happens to the tissue fragments the pathologist has chosen and given to the histologist for processing: the pieces are placed in little metal or plastic capsules which are perforated to allow circulation of the various fluids, and the capsules are loaded into a basket which is hung on the tissue processor — an Autotechnicon or similar machine. This instrument dips the basket into solution after solution, generally for an hour in each, throughout the night. First, there are generally two changes of formalin, then 80% alcohol, then two changes of 95% alcohol, and two more of 100% alcohol; then it goes through two or three changes of xylene, and finally two changes of melted paraffin. Since the tissue juices are basically water solutions, it would be impossible to replace them directly with melted paraffin, but by replacing water with alcohol, then alcohol with xylene, and xylene with paraffin, everything that was water in the tissue can finally be replaced with melted paraffin.

The tissue fragments are then placed into little containers and surrounded with paraffin which then cools and solidifies. The paraffin block with tissue is placed on a machine called a microtome for sectioning. The microtome will be discussed more fully in chapter eight, but it is one of the essential machines of pathology, whereby the tissue is cut into very thin slices. The microtome is very much like a butcher's meat slicer, but it cuts accurately at such a thinness that it would take three slices to be as thick as a red blood cell, and perhaps fifty or more slices to approach the thickness of a human hair. The slices made by the microtome adhere to each other at their edges, making a thin, delicate ribbon made up of paraffin and tissue slices. This ribbon is carefully spread on the surface of warm water to eliminate wrinkles, and then picked up on a glass slide and dried. Then the routine of the various solvents is reversed, to get rid of the paraffin and bring the tissue back to its watery state: the slide is dipped in xylene, alcohol, and into water, and then placed in a stain called hematoxylin, which is derived from the logwood tree of South America. After several rinses, it is counterstained with eosin, a coal-tar dye, then dipped repeatedly in the alcohol washes and in the xylene again. A drop of balsam is then placed on the tissue slice adhering to the slide, and a glass coverslip applied. (The balsam of today is a synthetic, but in former years, the clear, resinous, thick fluid from the blisters of the bark of the balsam tree was used.) Finally the slides are labeled and delivered to the pathologist.

Now the hard work starts; the pathologist examines the samples under the microscope, and he identifies the subtle differences caused by disease, in comparison to the normal appearances with which he is familiar. Often additional samples must be prepared, and new sections stained with other dyes to supplement the basic hematoxylin-and-eosin procedure (with which nearly all the routine sections are stained) because a particular problem cannot be solved using the standard dye. Whole books of special stains are in print, and many different procedures are often required.

Finally the pathologist settles down to complete his report on the autopsy. He has already dictated a description of the gross anatomic dissection and a page summarizing the clinical history. Now he completes a description of each tissue sample and organ he has examined through the microscope. At last the final diagnosis is stated, summarizing all of the anatomic abnormalities he has noted, grossly and microscopically, and the dictation is given to the typist. Perhaps a month after the start of the autopsy, the typing is ready for the pathologist to review and sign, and the case is completed.

Well, not quite completed. The report must be given to the

hospital record room to be attached to the hospital chart of the deceased, and a copy is given to the doctor who attended the patient before the death so he can inform the family about the autopsy findings. It is better to have the attending physician do this, rather than the pathologist, because he, at least theoretically, knows the family and can therefore more readily answer their questions and couch his answers in terms that the family can best understand. Copies of the autopsy report must be given to the medical examiner in medical-legal cases. And the clerks must now undertake the chore of coding the diagnoses so that the case can be cross-indexed with other cases of the same disease. There are innumerable details to take care of.

Even then, the pathologist is not through; he must be ready to discuss the case at clinical service meetings and at hospital death conferences because every death is followed up in order to further the study of disease and of how it may be treated more successfully. In medical-legal cases, court appearances and hearings are yet to come.

All in all, the autopsy procedure is a long and difficult process, requiring highly trained personnel and expensive equipment. It should not be difficult to understand why it is expensive, and the expense side of autopsy is discussed further in chapter sixteen. But the results obtained are very important to society, and worth every bit of the time and trouble.

CHAPTER FOUR

THE AUTOPSY REPORT

On the next pages, I will go through a typical autopsy report. This case is a fictional composite of the features of a number of cases. It is not too complicated, and the diseases diagnosed could easily have happened to one person. Many cases are much more complicated and others could be much simpler. I have tried to construct a reasonable case, which illustrates a number of aspects of the autopsy report.

The standard disclaimer of "any resemblance of any actual person living or dead is purely coincidental" must be modified by striking out the word "living," but it otherwise applies here.

One might find a longer and more detailed autopsy report on a case very much like this one, but some pathologists would make a shorter, sketchy report. The style here is modified teaching hospital style, as far as length and detail is concerned. Items of style will vary widely from hospital to hospital, but there is one convention that is accepted everywhere: the report, except for the clinical history summary, is written in the present tense. Even when the narrative style used here is replaced by single-word or phrase reporting, the present tense is used.

The non-narrative autopsy report is a checklist in which the prosector may insert a word or phrase on a printed form, and write in the figures for the weights and measurements. In theory, any time a narrative report is needed, it can be written by turning the checklist information into sentences. This saves a lot of time, but I know from experience that it is virtually impossible to reconstruct all of the details from the checklist, and that the

Autopsy No. A84-159 Hospital No. N65578

Central New England Medical Center
Renfield, Massachusetts

AUTOPSY REPORT

Name Johnson, Charles Age 59 Sex M Race W

Date of Admission 4-25 19 84 Date of Death 5-22 19 84

Clinical Service Med II Attending Doctor B. Ahearn

Date of Autopsy 5-22 19 84 at 2:30 p.m.

Staff Pathologist Dr. Burgess Prosector Dr. Murphy

Permission from Miss Mary Johnson Relationship Daughter

Restrictions None

FINAL DIAGNOSIS

Primary

Generalized arteriosclerosis, especially of coronary and renal arteries and aorta
Aneurysm, abdominal aorta
Healed and healing myocardial infarct, anterior wall of left ventricle, with acute extension to lateral wall
Healed surgical scar of chest with coronary bypass, anterior descending and circumflex coronary arteries
Surgical scars of legs, bilaterally (vein donor sites)
Pulmonary emphysema, marked, with fibrosis
Old infarcts of lungs, lower lobes bilaterally
Fibrous pleural adhesions
THROMBLSIS OF ANTERIOR CORONARY BYPASS
THROMBOSIS OF LEG VEINS WITH THROMBOEMBOLIC OCCLUSION OF PULMONARY ARTERIES, BILATERALLY
Acute pulmonary edema

Subsidiary

Old healed pulmonary tuberculosis, left upper lobe of lung
Small-cell carcinoma, right upper lobe bronchus
Metastatic small-cell carcinoma, two mediastinal lymph nodes
Healed surgical scar of abdomen, with absence of appendix.
Fibrous peritoneal adhesions
Benign prostatic hypertrophy

Date of dictation: 6-5-84
Date of transcription: 6-16-84

Samuel B. Burgess, M.D.
Samuel B. Burgess, M.D., Pathologist

Figure 1

whole flavor of the autopsy can thus be lost. There is nothing that replaces the narrative style of report, dictated promptly after, or even during, the autopsy. The best reports are done from notes; and are done immediately after the autopsy procedure, while seated comfortably at a desk with a minimum of distraction.

In this chapter, we present a typical autopsy report is presented on each left-hand page, while the facing right-hand page is a commentary on that particular page. I hope, in this presentation, to make clear some of the technical terms, and some of the implications of the statements made. These implications should not be any problem to the physician reading the report, but others without medical school training will probably need some of the nuances explained.

The page shown in Figure 1 is called the Face Sheet. It carries the information which identifies the patient and the details which permit the establishment of various files. The entire report will be sent to the record room, filed under the Hospital Number at the upper right of the page. This file will be available in perpetuity, microfilmed after two or three years. These records are closely guarded, and the record room librarian must have authorization by the doctor and the patient's family, or a court order, to show the record to anyone.

At the upper left is the laboratory serial number of the autopsy. The prefix "A" indicates Autopsy; surgical pathology records are filed under"S," and the cytology records under "P" (for the cancer smear technique first described by George Papanicolaou). The typed records of these three groups are easy to distinguish, but the glass slides for microscopic study are very similar in appearance, hence the prefixes. The laboratory copy of these reports will be bound in a volume as permanent laboratory record.

A copy of the report is sent to the doctor who cared for the patient so he will have the information to talk to the family of the deceased. Generally, the report is not given to the family, since technical details and professional jargon are likely to confuse. The attending doctor generally talks with the family, or writes a letter to summarize the findings, but sometimes the pathologist will talk or write to them at his request.

The details above the *Final Diagnosis* line are self-explanatory. Age, sex and race are recorded to aid anyone who wants to

A84-159

CLINICAL HISTORY

This 59-year-old white male housepainter entered the Local Community Hospital 27 days prior to death, complaining of malaise, fever, and shortness of breath. He had been in good health until three years earlier, when he fell from a ladder and suffered a broken leg. While hospitalized following this accident, he had repeated episodes of syncope, confusion, chest pain, and breathlessness. but recovered without specific therapy within several weeks and returned to work, ignoring gradually increasing angina. He missed repeated follow-up appointments with his family doctor. One year prior to his final admission, he developed severe anterior chest pain, with disphoresis and anxiety, and was again hospitalized at Local Community Hospital, where EKG showed anterior myocardial infarction. Following recovery from this, cardiac angiography demonstrated marked narrowing of the enterior descending and circumflex branches of the left coronary artery, and he was transferred to C.N.E. Medical Center. Coronary bypass of the two vessels was carried out. Following discharge, he was much improved, and returned to work without angina until his final episode.

The patient was a known heavy smoker (2½ packs of cigarettes per day) but used alcohol only occasionally. His parentage was Scandinavian and English. His parents died many year before', of unknown causes. Two sisters are living and well. His wife died of tuberculosis, ten year before the final admission.

The patient was transferred here from Local Community Hospital 24 hours after admission there, with no specific therapy having been undertaken. On admission here, he was a well-developed and well-nourished white male in moderate distress, complaining of shortness of breath. Cardiac auscultation showed regular sinus rhythm with occasional extrasystoles and a grade 2 mitral systolic murmur. Lungs showed questionable dullnuss in the upper lung fields, with expiratory rales. The abdomen was slightly distended, with a well-healed scar of old appendectomy. There was slight ankle edema, and questionable cyanosis of the nailbeds. Neurological examination and other findings were within normal limits.

Laboratory studies showed WBC of 12,500, with 68% polys, 5% bands, 24% lymphs, 2% eos, and 1% monos. Chemistry profile was normal except BUN of 30 mgm% and uric acid of 9 mgm%. Cardiac enzymes were consistant with acute myocardial infarction. EKG was interpreted as showing old myocardial infarct of the anterior wall, with acute extension. Sputum cultures grew out staphylococcus and E. coli.

The patient was treated with heparin, and with erythromycin and later cephalosporin versus the mixed bacterial infection. EKG showed no apparent progression of the infarction, and the patient was transferred from the intensive care unit, and permitted to ambulate. He was observed to collapse suddenly, with marked hyperpnea, and expired in spite of vigorous attempts at resuscitation.

Figure 2

identify a particular group of cases for statistical purposes. The resident, Dr. Murphy, a pathologist in training, performed the autopsy, and Dr. Burgess has attended the autopsy and reviewed the tissue sections under the microscope. Dr. Burgess is the pathologist who supervised this case and studied the completed report before signing; and he holds the ultimate legal and professional responsibility for the case.

This autopsy was performed the same day as the death. Sometimes, if the death has been in the evening, it might be done the next morning. The conscientious pathology department wants to get the examination done as quickly as possible, as seen in chapter eleven.

The rest of the face sheet lists the final diagnosis. I will discuss the details step by step, and at the end of the chapter.

The pathologist's summary is not the same as the complete, detailed summary the attending doctor writes upon hospital discharge. The pathologist tries to give a general overview of the case, but if someone needs a detailed study, he should go to the hospital records. The pathologist summarizes only those items which will help the reader understand the case.

This clinical history (Figure 2) has some interesting features which raise many questions — only a few of which can be answered by the autopsy. The patient entered with apparent pneumonia, but at his death, this had been cured. His occupation as house painter suggests exposure to chemicals, but we'll see that this was not the cause of death. His first hospitalization was for a broken leg, but did he fall from the ladder because disease caused him to faint?

Clearly, he had heart disease before his first hospitalization, but he chose to ignore it, and after discharge from the hospital, he was careless in taking care of himself. But finally, increasing heart disease could not be ignored, and he accepted a coronary bypass operation which helped him a great deal.

His smoking has a direct bearing on his disease since it clearly causes, not only lung cancer, but heart disease and emphysema, among other diseases. His ethnic origin is included to suggest elimination of those diseases that run in some racial groups, such as thalassemia, or Buerger's disease. His exposure to his wife's tuberculosis was related to his disease, but not to his death.

Of course, a complete report would include much more detail in the physical examination and laboratory findings, but the prosector rightly judged that these were not necessary to under-

A84-159

EXTERNAL EXAMINATION

The body is that of a well-developed, well-nourished white male of about the stated age of 59, measuring 176 cm. in length, and weighing approximately 80 kg. There is no apparent rigor of the extremities, and no dependant mottling of the body. There is no unusual pigmentation or icterus of the skin. There is no gross deformity of the body, and no sign of external trauma. Surgical scars are described below.

HEAD - The head is symmetrical and semi-bald, with a rim of grey hair. The scalp is clean

EYES - The eyes show pupils that are round, equal, and regular, and measure 4 mm. The irides are grey. The sclerae are clear, with no icterus.

NOSE - The nose shows no external deformity. The nares are clear.

MOUTH - The lips and tongue present the usual appearance. The teeth are carious and dirty, with several teeth missing. The oropharynx is clear.

NECK - The neck shows no masses or other unusual finding.

THORAX - The thorax is symmetrical. There is a healed operative scar 25 cm. in length, vertically placed in the midline, consistant with previous coronary bypass surgery. There is no nodulation or ulceration of this scar. The breasts are normal male.

ABDOMEN - The abdomen is rounded and symmetrical, with no masses or other unusual finding on palpation. There is a healed operative scar of the right lower quadrant, consistant with previous appendectomy.

GENITALIA - The genitalia are normal adult male.

EXTREMITIES - The extremities show no apparent fracture or deformity. There are healed operative scars of the inner aspect of both thighs, mearsuring 30 cm. on the left and 25 cm. on the right, consistant with removal of vein segemnts as donor tissue for coronary bypass. There is slight pitting edema of the ankles bilaterally, and slight cyanosis of the nailbeds. There is no clubbing of fingers.

INTERNAL EXAMINATION

ABDOMINAL CAVITY - The body is opened through the usual Y-shaped incision, revealing an adipose layer 3.5 cm. in thickness, and well-developed muscular layer. The peritoneum is incised, revealing the abdominal organs in their usual relationship, and no unusual collection of fluid. There are scattered dense fibrous adhesions in the right lower quadrant involving the small and large intestine in the area of the surgical scar seen externally. The appendix is absent, and the stump of the appendix is well-healed. The liver edge projects 5 cm. below the xyphoid process, but is above the costal margin elsewhere. The dome of the diaphragm is at the level of the fifth intercostal space bilaterally.

Figure 3

stand the case. And likewise, many of the details of his hospital course are left out; all the medications he was given aren't listed, only the heparin, designed to prevent thrombosis of the coronary arteries (though it wasn't successful), and the antibiotics which cleared his pneumonia.

In fact, he was doing very well, and was approaching discharge when he died suddenly, as noted on the face sheet, of a pulmonary embolism from the thrombosed leg veins. This is not an uncommon cause of death, and one of the hardest to anticipate and prevent, since it gives no symptoms before the final event.

If this patient had not been autopsied, I'll bet he would have been signed out as a heart attack.

Figure 3, illustrates where the description of the actual gross autopsy begins. Before any incision with the scalpel, the external appearance of the body is studied and recorded. The prosector measures the body, and estimates the weight unless the autopsy room has facilities for actually weighing the body. Although many laboratories still record these figures in English units, there is a growing tendency to use metric units throughout.

The conscientious prosector not only looks at the body on the table, he rolls it up on one side and examines the back. I can think of only one time that I would have missed a finding by not examining the back, but I did it throughout my career to make sure. In the case of a very heavy body, the diener assists the pathologist in rolling the body over. The diener, at this point in the autopsy, has already laid out the various instruments and removed the shroud which has covered the body in its journey from the hospital ward, and he stands ready to assist the prosector by lifting, pulling, and such work. Any time he is not so occupied, he should be standing ready to wipe up little spills of blood, and keeping the instruments clean and ready.

The external appearance is carefully described, and all old operative and traumatic scars are recorded, even if they are years old and not in any way related to the final disease. One thing I note in this record is that the ears have not been examined, or at least, been skipped in the description; this should have been included, but it does not detract from the autopsy. It only gives the impression that the prosector was not as careful as he should have been. Since I signed this case, that means me, as well!

A84-159

THORACIC CAVITY - The sternal triangle is removed, revealing the thoracic organs in their usual relationship, and no unusual collection of fluid. The sternum is sutured with eight wire loops, and there are dense fibrous adhesions of the lung bilaterally to the anterior thoracic cage, consistant with previous operative intervention. The posterior and lateral surfaces of the lungs show no adhesions.

PERICARDIAL CAVITY - The pericardial cavity is obliterated by dense fibrous adhesions, and the pericardial membrane is missing over the anterior portion. The right lung is adherant to the e½icardium in this area.

HEART - The heart weighs 400 grams. The external surface shows multiple tags of fibrous adhesions. There is the usual amount of subepicardial fat. The external examination reveals an anterior bypass replacing the descending coronary artery, and a second bypass replacing a portion of the circumflex branch. These originate in the ascending aorta, 2.0 cm. distal to the normal coronary orfices. The circumflex bypass is soft and patent, but the descending graft is firm and shows occlusion by thrombus on cut surface, for 3.0 cm. near its midpoint. Cut surfaces of the myocardium measure 0.3 cm. in the right ventricle, and 1.8 cm. in the left ventricle. There is an area of marked thinning and replacement of the myocardial tissue by fibrous tissue in the anterior wall, 5.0 cm. in diameter and reaching onto the apical area. The lateral wall shows deep-red mottling and an area of brown softening adjacent to the old fibrous area. The posterior and septal walls are unremarkable, and the endocardium is smooth, with no adherant mural thrombus. There is slight dilatation of the left ventricle. The valvular circumferences are as follows: tricuspid 14.0 cm., pulmonic 8.0 cm., aortic 7.5 cm., mitral 10.5 cm.; there is no apparent stenosis or insufficiency of any of the valves. The great vessels arise in their usual relationship, and the only abnormality is the bypass vessels sutured into the ascending aorta as described above. The atrial appendages are free of clot. The coronary arteries are followed by multiple section, and show very marked sclerotic narrowing throughout, with pin-point lumen in many areas, and complete occlusion of the anterior descending and circumflex branches, where the bypass grafts are placed.

LUNGS - The right lung weighs 850 grams; the left lung weighs 695 grams. The external surface os each shows multiple tags of dense fibrous adhesions. There is moderate emphysematous change, with fibrosis in the apices bilaterally, and with a sense of marked density in the left apex. No discrete masses are palpated. Cut surface of the right lung reveals a mass 2.5 cm. in diameter, apparently arising from the right upper lobe bronchus 3.0 cm. from the carina, with irregular, granular tissue replacing the smooth lining of the bronchus over an area 1.0 by 1.5 cm. Cut surface of the left apex shows dense fibrous tissue, with a 1.2 cm. nodule of light-grey tissue consistant with old tuberculoma. Elsewhere, the cut surfaces exude abundant bloody, frothy fluid, with no apparent consolidation, abscess, or other lesion. A coarse emphysematous pattern is found throughout. The pulmonary arteries are completely occluded by thrombotic material which does not conform to the shape of the pulmonary vessels; there is no apparent organization of these clots. The bronchi, except in the area of tumor described, are unremarkable throughout. The lymph nodes of the mediastinum are described below.

Figure 4

The last paragraph begins the actual cutting part of the autopsy. The Y-shaped incision begins from each shoulder and joins over the xiphoid process (the lower end of the breastbone), and continues as a single cut down over the abdomen to the level of the pubic bone. The various layers of the abdominal wall are examined before the incision into the abdominal cavity, then the abdominal cavity is examined, both visually and by manual exploration, and any abnormality recorded. Here, there is no abnormality, and all of the organs are found to be present, except the appendix — which has been removed some time in the past, and the operation has resulted in the formation of fibrous adhesions, not an unusual consequence of any surgical operation involving the abdominal viscera.

Next the thoracic cavity is explored (Figure 4), and for this, the ribs are cut up each side, and removed with the breastbone. Again, there are fibrous adhesions; these might have resulted from old pleurisy, but I think they probably came from small lung infarcts when he fell from the ladder. His leg fracture allowed small fragments of bone marrow to enter the veins and travel to the lungs, blocking arteries and killing the lung tissue. The fibrous adhesions of the pericardial cavity, the sac in which the heart normally lies free and movable except for its blood-vessel attachments at the upper end, clearly resulted from the operation for coronary bypass. Some of the pericardial wall had to be removed, and the right lung is adherent in this area.

The heart is removed by cutting the large arteries and veins, and is weighed. In this case, the weight is above normal, and the wall of the left ventricle is thicker than normal; these findings are consistent with high blood pressure, and represent a normal response of the heart to the load that is imposed. The heart must, in such a circumstance, either hypertrophy or fail.

The coronary bypass grafts are noted to be in place, and significantly, the anterior bypass is filled with clot. When the muscle is cut across, there is fresh necrosis of the lateral wall near the old scar from his heart attack. The coronary arteries, as expected, are very hardened and blocked. Several routine findings are recorded, such as the size of the four valves of the heart. In this case, these measurements are entirely normal, but if there had been old rheumatic disease, one or more valves might have been thickened and narrowed.

A84-159

LIVER - The liver weighs 1750 grams. The external surface is deep reddish-brown and smooth. There is moderate rounding of the liver edge. The cut surface exudes abundant bloody fluid. There is no apparent abscess, tumor, or other abnormality. The portal vein presents the usual appearance. The gall bladder is 9.2 cm. in length and 3.0 cm. in diameter. The external surface is smooth. The cut organ shows clear green bile, with no calculi or other unusual finding. The bile ducts are unremarkable; the common bile duct empties into the duodenum independently from the pancreatic duct.

SPLEEN - The spleen weighs 120 grams. The external surface is deep reddish-grey and smooth. Cut surfces show deep red, homogeneous tissue, with no apparent infarct or other lesion.

PANSREAS - The pancreas weighs 110 grams. The external shape is unremarkable. Cut surfaces show the usual pinkish-grey, lobulated tissue, with no apparent tumor, fibrosis, or other abnormality. The pancreatic duct is unremarkable.

ADRENALS - The adrenals together weigh 18 grams. Their external shape is unremarkable. Cut surfaces show the usual tan cortex and grey medulla, with no hemorrhage, tumor, or other lesion.

GENITO-URINARY SYSTEM - The right kidney weighs 160 grams; the left kidney weighs 170 grams. The capsule is stripped with ease from each, revealing a finely granular surface, with no depressed scars. Cut surfaces show moderate narrowing of the renal parenchyma, and moderate loss of cortico-medullary differentiation. There is no cyst formation or tumor. The renal pelves present the usual appearance. The ureters are unremarkable. The bladder wall is somewhat thickened, but the lining is smooth, with no trabeculation. The prostate is approximately three times normal size, but is smooth and symmetrical. The testicles present the usual appearance throughout.

GASTRO-INTESTINAL SYSTEM - The esophagus and stomach present the usual appearance, with no apparent ulceration, tumor, or other abnormality. The stomach contains a small amount of partially-digested food and cloudy grey fluid; there are no pill-remanents or other unusual contents. The small intestine is unremarkable in its entire extent, with no apparent ulcer or obstruction. The large intestine contains a large amount of formed, brown stool in the distal portions, but no apparent lesion. The appendix is surgically absent, and the stump of appendix is well-healed.

LYMPH NODES - Ten lymph nodes of the mediastinum are identified, and the two largest of these, each measuring 0.9 cm., show nodules of firm grey tumor tissue. The other lymph nodes show soft pink cut surfaces. There is no apparent lymphadenopathy elsewhere.

Figure 5

The lungs are removed and weighed. Immediately seen is the cause of death, although the finding is recorded at the end of the paragraph; the pulmonary arteries are completely plugged by blood clot, and these clots are not the same shape as the pulmonary artery, showing that they formed elsewhere, in this case, in the veins of the leg, where they broke loose and floated through the bloodstream until they plugged the pulmonary artery, bringing the whole circulation of blood to a halt.

The coarse emphysema seen throughout the lungs is the result of the patient's long-term smoking. Emphysema kills five or six people for every cancer death from smoking.

The old focus of tuberculosis in the left lung is noted, and above all, the tobacco-caused cancer, which was not related to his death, but would have killed him soon, if the embolism hadn't.

The remainder of the abdominal organs are now described (Figure 5) in the usual orderly fashion. The spleen, pancreas, and adrenals are completely normal. The liver, though, is congested, apparently as a consequence of the stoppage of the circulation by the pulmonary emboli, otherwise, the liver, too, is normal, as is the gallbladder. It is customary to note the arrangements of the bile ducts and the portal vein; the point of emptying of the common bile duct into the duodenum is of interest, because, in a few cases, it is joined by the pancreatic duct, and this arrangement can lead to acute pancreatitis if a stone gets stuck in the bile duct.

The kidneys, on the other hand, do show some disease. There is blood vessel disease which has some implications for the patient. A few of the operating units of the kidney (the nephrons) are replaced by scar tissue, and this is the consequence of sclerosis of the arterial supply. The narrowing of the arteries has also caused the kidney cells to overproduce a hormonal substance called renin, which stimulates the capillaries throughout the body into contracting, and results in high blood pressure. It would appear almost as if the kidney was sending this signal to increase the blood pressure, and this has had its effect elsewhere; the heart, as previously noted, has had to develop more muscle. All in all, this patient's elevation of blood pressure would not have been very great, and in the clinical history it was not even mentioned, so it must have been slight.

The stomach and intestines fall within normal limits. The patient died suddenly, having eaten a meal (apparently breakfast according to the timing in this case) so some food is noted to be in the stomach. But there is no ulcer, a disease quite common among house painters for reasons unknown, and there is no cancer of the stomach. The prosector has opened the entire small

A84-159

NECK ORGANS - The esophagus and trachea are midline, and show no apparent abnormality. The thyroid weighs 14 grams, and is symmetrical, with deep pink cut surfaces, and no apparent nodulation. The larynx presents the usual appearance.

BLOOD VESSELS - The thoracic aorta shows fairly marked sclerosis, with egg-shell calcification, but no mural thrombus. The abdominal aorta is even more sclerotic, and there is aneurysmal dilatation of the right lateral wall, from 4 cm. distal to the renal arteries to the bifurcation. This bulge shows moderate calcification of the wall, and there is a patch of adherant mural thrombus 1.5 cm. in thickness lying in the aneurysm; this is firmly attached. The medium sized arteries are moderatly sclerotic, but show no apparent occlusion. The thrombo-embolic occlusion of the pulmonary arteris is described above. The veins present the usual appearance in all areas except the upper legs, where there is absence of portions of the saphenous veins bilaterally, the cut ends of which are well tied off, with no hemorrhage. A small amount of thrombotic material is found proximal to the proximal line of excision. The femoral vien is dissected, and shows thrombus formation in the distal portions; it is obvious that this is the site of origin of the thrombo-embolism.

SKELETAL SYSTEM - The skeletal system shows no fracture, deformity, or other lesion. The vertebral bone marrow presents the usual appearance.

CRANIAL CONTENTS - The scalp is reflected and the calvarium opened in the usual manner, revealing no apparent lesion. The scalp is thicker than usual, measuring 1.9 cm. The bone of the calvarium is likewise quite thick, averaging 1.1 cm. over the major portion of the skull. The meninges show no apparent clouding or hemorrhage. There is the usual amount of cerebro-spinal fluid, which is colorless and clear. The brain is removed and weighs 1565 grams. The cerebral hemispheres are symmetrical, and there is no apparent flattening of gyri or widening of sulci. The base of brain presents the usual appearance throughout, and the vessels of the Circle of Willis show moderate sclerosis, but no apparent occlusion. The pons, medulla, and cerebellum are symmetrical and show no abnormality. The cut end of spinal cord shows the usual appearance. The brain is sectioned at 1.0 cm. intervals, revealing slight narrowing of the grey matter of the cerebral hemispheres. The underlying white matter shows no cyst formation, hemorrhage, or other lesion. The putamen and globus pallidus are of average appearance, and the caudate nucleus and thalmus are likewise of average appearance. The ventricles are of average proportions throughout, and contain clear fluid. Cut surfaces of the brain stem show no tumor, cyst formation, hemorrhage or other lesion, and cut surfaces of the cerebellum are similarly unremarkable. Internal examination of the bony skull show no evidence of fracture or other lesion. The pituitary is of average appearance.

Figure 6

and large intestine looking for cancer, ulcer, diverticulitis, or some other disease, and has found none.

Among the lymph nodes there are only two of interest; these lie in the mediastinum (the area between the two lungs where the trachea, the main-stem bronchi, and the great vessels [the arch of the aorta and the two vena cava structures] are located). The two lymph nodes lie in the drainage of the right lung, and the small cancer there has already extended to them. Even if the small cancer had been discovered, the patient would not have been curable by surgery.

The page shown in Figure 6 completes the gross examination. The prosector is recording the last details of the main body cavity, and examining the brain cavity. He explores the neck for any abnormality and finds none; the thyroid appears just about normal, and the larynx is without disease.

The blood vessels, which have been examined along with the other organs, are described in one paragraph for orderly presentation; here the prosector indeed finds disease. The arterial system is quite sclerotic, and the aorta has eggshell calcification. This process increases on down the aorta, and below the arteries to the kidneys the wall is so weak that it has started to balloon outward. Sometimes these arteriosclerotic aneurysms can burst, causing extensive bleeding into the tissues of the flanks and even an abdominal cavity filled with blood, and resulting in sudden death. In this case, the bulge is small, and the wall has become thickened by a blood clot firmly attached to the lining of the bulge.

The veins are of interest for two reasons. First, portions of the saphenous veins of the upper leg have been removed by the surgeon to use as a graft in his coronary bypass operation. Although veins are thin-walled and lack a muscular coat, they can be used successfully to bypass sclerotic arteries for short distances. The saphenous veins can be removed and their function can be carried out by the deeper veins, the femorals. But second, in this case, the femoral vein had become thrombosed, probably because of the inactivity of the patient lying in bed. When he started to walk around, this clot became dislodged and it traveled to his lungs, causing his death. Sometimes the entire clot dislodges, but here, there was a small amount of clot remaining in the femoral vein.

The examination of the head completes the gross autopsy. Sometimes the diener incises and strips the scalp, and saws the bone of the head to help the prosector, but any abnormalities must be noted on the way in, as with the trunk incision. In this case everything is normal. The brain weight is about what it

A84-159

MICROSCOPIC DESCRIPTION

HEART - Section of the myocardium of the anterior wall shows very extensive replacement of myocardial cells by dense fibrous tissue. The lateral wall shows necrosis of muscle cells, and infiltration of polymorphonuclear leukocytes and extravasation of erythrocytes. The endocardium is unremarkable, and the base of mitral valve shows no lesion. Sections of coronary arteries show marked sclerosis, with apparent complete occlusion of the lumen by cholesterol and semi-calcified debris. Section of the anterior-descending bypass segment shows complete occlusion by thrombus, with very early organizational ingrowth of fibroblasts at its edges. Epicardial layers are thickened, with fibroblastic activity in many areas.

LUNGS - Sections from all areas show very marked emphysematous change, with marked interstitial fibrosis. Alveolar walls are extensively destroyed, and large, air-containing spaces are present. Many other alveolar spaces contain proteinaceous fluid, but there is no evidence of any inflammatory infiltrate or pneumonic consolidation. Moderate interstitial lymphocytosis is noted. Section from the left upper lobe show very marked fibrosis, with a focal area of caseous necrosis, and two giant-cells of the Langhans type. Acid-fast stain of this area confirms the presence of tubercle bacilli. There is moderate palis-sading of epitheleoid cells around this area of necrosis. Section of the nodule attached to the right-upper-lobe bronchus shows the presence of malignant tumor; the tumor cells are small and highly hyperchromatic, with very scanty cytoplasm. Occasional larger cells are present, and occasional mitoses are identified, some of which are atypical. Many other mitoses are apparently concealed by the hyperchromatic nuclear material. The center of the tumor nodule shows moderate necrosis. The tumor tends to infiltrate the surrounding pulmonary parenchyma, and probable lymph-channel invasion is noted. The tumor is closely associated with the bronchial epithelium in several areas, and the bronchi outside the area of tumor show patches of squamous metaplasia, with lymphocytic infiltration of their walls. Sections of the lower lobes of lungs bilaterally show circumscribed areas of old dense fibrosis, consistant with old healed pulmonary infarcts. There is fairly marked fluid deposition in the lower lobes, but no inflammatory change. Section of the material within the main pul-monary artery branches bilaterally show unorganized thrombotic material.

LIVER - Section shows moderate congestion of the hepatic sinusoids and central veins. The portal areas show no increased fibrosis; and no inflammatory infiltrate. There is very slight fatty metamorphosis of the liver cord cells in the peri-portal areas. The vessels and bile duct branches within the portal areas show no duplication or other lesion. No malignant tumor is present at the several levels examined.

GALL BLADDER - Sections show no apparent thickening of the gall bladder wall, and no fusion of plicae. There is no apparent inflammation, and no crypt formation.

Figure 7

should be, and the only abnormality noted in the entire head examination is the moderate sclerosis (hardening) of the Circle of Willis, a circle of arteries at the base of the brain. It is thrombosis (clotting) or rupture in this circle or its branches which results in a stroke, since the main blood supply of the brain passes through here, but our patient had neither rupture nor thrombosis.

The microscopic examination (Figure 7) follows a couple of weeks after the gross autopsy. The body has been turned over to the undertaker, with a provisional diagnosis, which allows a death certificate to be written. During the gross autopsy the prosector has selected small bits of tissues to be made into slides for the microscope by the histologist. The prosector has taken preliminary looks at them and ordered any additional slides or special stains he needs to understand the case. He's now ready to write the description of the microscopic examination, and the final diagnosis.

In the heart, as expected, dense fibrous scar is found replacing the heart muscle in the anterior wall of the left ventricle; this was his old heart attack. And again as expected, the extension of the heart attack to a new area in the lateral wall is evidenced by dead tissue. There are no surprises in the heart; the coronary bypass is plugged by clot, which caused the final heart attack. The early ingrowth of fibroblasts indicates that this blockage happened several days before his death. His new heart attack was "silent," that is, it occurred without the usual chest pain.

The lungs are a museum of pathology. There is advanced emphysema with fibrosis caused by long-term smoking. And also because of smoking, there is a small cancer of the right lung, arising from the bronchus near the root of the lung ; this is the common location for a smoker's cancer, and this location at the root makes surgery impossible. These cancers are usually out of control by the time they are discovered. In the lung there is also a tuberculoma: an area of necrosis surrounded by a characteristic arrangement of epithelioid cells and Langhans' giant cells, and special stains demonstrate the tubercle bacillus, the *Mycobacterium tuberculosis*.

The plugging of the pulmonary artery is confirmed by the tissue samples, which provide permanent documentation of the clot seen at the gross autopsy. The abundant fluid which was seen grossly, is documented by the proteinaceous material on the slide.

The examination of the liver and the gallbladder gives a long list of findings, none significant except for the congestion

A84-159

SPLEEN - Sections show very marked congestion of the splenic parenchyma. There is no apparent germanitive activity in the small malpighian bodies. The arterioles show slight hyaline sclerosis. There is no inflammation or infarction.

PANCREAS - Sections show well-formed digestive glandular elements, with no apparent fibrosis, inflammation, or other abnormality. The endocrine islands present the usual appearance throughout. The pancreatic duct lining is unremarkable.

ADRENALS - Sections of the adrenals bilaterally show abundant cortical tissue, with medullary elements of average appearance. The cortical cells are arranged in the usual fashion. There is no apparent inflammation, tumor, or hemorrhage.

KIDNEYS - Sections of the cortical portions bilaterally show replacement of scattered glomeruli by dense fibrous scar. Other glomeruli are well-formed and unremarkable. The arterioles of many glomeruli show moderate hyaline sclerosis, but no apparent occlusion. Larger arterial branches show thickening of their walls, with cholesterol deposition and focal calcification, but no apparent occclusion. The tubular elements of the cortical and medullary layers are replaced in scattered areas by fibrous tissue. The tubular epithelium is well-preserved and unremarkable. The collecting system shows no lesion, and the renal pelvic epithelium presents the usual appearance, with no inflammation or other lesion.

PROSTATE - Sections of the prostate show multiple nodules of large glands lined by cuboidal epithelium, but no evidence of small-gland formation, and no apparent malignant change. Focal areas show lymphocytic infiltration, but there is no apparent acute inflammation. Adjacent bladder-wall sectionsshow moderate hypertrophy of the muscular wall, and unremarkable trnasitional epithelium.

THYROID - Sections show large acini with abundant colloid material, often showing vacuolization of the edges. There is no apparent nodule formation, and no malignant change.

BRAIN - Sections are examined representing cerebral cortex, putamen and globus pallidus, thalmus, pons, cerebellum, and medulla. There is no apparent gliosis, and no inflammation or abcess formation. The cortical nerve cells present the usual appearance, and the supporting structures are unremarkable. The grey matter of the basal ganglia shows no apparent lesion. The ependymal tissue is unremarkable. There is no evidence of malignant change at any point.

Figure 8

of the liver tissue. Most of the negative findings are listed just to rule out a number of specific diseases.

The spleen shows some congestion which was not noted in the gross examination, but this is not surprising, since the liver, with its similar blood supply, is congested. The hyaline sclerosis of the arterioles is quite common, and associated with aging.

The pancreas and the adrenals are entirely normal, as was expected. The endocrine islands of the pancreas are the small areas of tissue that produce insulin to control diabetes, and this patient was not diabetic. The remainder of the pancreas produces digestive enzymes. The adrenal cortex produces many hormones, including cortisone and sex hormones; the medulla produces the emergency hormone familiarly known as adrenalin; the patient had no problems in this area.

The kidneys show the scarring that were suggested by the gross examination. There is no inflammation or tumor, but there is disease of the blood vessels which is associated with the kidney hormone which leads to hypertension, as discussed above. The arteries are somewhat sclerotic, and the tiny arterioles, as they enter the glomeruli (the filtration units of kidney), are narrowed by hyaline sclerosis, which is a different process from arteriosclerosis. Perhaps there should be another diagnosis on the face sheet, of arteriolonephronsclerosis.

The patient shows benign hypertrophy of the prostate, a common finding in older men. Small cancers of the prostate are also often found among older men, but not here — at least in the samples examined. Perhaps if fifty or sixty samples had been taken, a small cancer might have been found, but cost-benefit analysis would not justify it.

A lot of sections were taken at various places in the brain tissue, so as to give a general overview of anything that might be going on, but each one of the sections examined shows only normal appearances. This is often the case in the general run of autopsies; the brain, as important as it is, is only occasionally the site of significant disease. Most people die with apparently normal brains.

Returning to the face sheet and considering what this autopsy has shown, here is the prosector's list of diagnoses:

Generalized arteriosclerosis, especially of coronary and renal arteries and aorta
Aneurysm, abdominal aorta
Healed and healing myocardial infarct, anterior wall of left ventricle, with acute extension to lateral wall.
Healed surgical scar of chest with coronary bypass, anterior descending and circumflex coronaries

Surgical scars of legs (vein donor sites)
Pulmonary emphysema, marked with fibrosis
Old infarcts of lungs, lower lobes bilaterally
Fibrous pleural adhesions
THROMBOSIS ANTERIOR CORONARY BYPASS
THROMBOSIS OF LEG VEINS WITH THROMBO-EMBOLIC OCCLUSION OF PULMONARY ARTERIES, BILATERALLY
Acute pulmonary edema

These are the diagnoses which are related in one way or another to the cause of death. They are arranged in a rough chronological order, with the oldest disease first, so the person reading the report will get a rough idea of the sequence of events as they occurred. Incidentally, the pulmonary emphysema probably should have been listed earlier, and the old infarcts of lungs, as well. The doctor making out the death certificate has to write it in the opposite order, since the standard death certificates used by all states ask for the immediate cause, followed by "due to" and again "due to" (for subsidiary cause), so this case would appear on the death certificate as *"Pulmonary embolism, due to thrombosis of leg veins, due to generalized arteriosclerosis,"* which does not give a really good picture of the case.

Now, here are the subsidiary diagnoses:

Old healed pulmonary tuberculosis, left upper lobe of lung
Small cell carcinoma, right upper lobe bronchus
Metastatic tumor, two mediastinal lymph nodes
Healed surgical scar of abdomen, with absence of appendix
Fibrous peritoneal adhesions
Benign prostatic hypertrophy

Some of these diagnoses are highly significant. It would be hard to argue that the lung cancer with extension to local lymph nodes is not important, and likewise the tuberculosis. But *subsidiary* does not mean unimportant, it merely means that these diseases — important as they are to the patient, the patient's family, and to society generally — did not operate as part of the mechanism which produced the patient's death. The cancer is very important as another addition to the long statistical proof that smoking causes cancer; there's no compelling evidence that this particular cancer was caused by smoking, but taken with all the other cases, it works out that it's about a ninety-five percent certainty that it was. The pattern is repeated too many times to suggest that the vast bulk of these cancers are not caused by smoking.

At the bottom of the face sheet the date of dictation is recorded; this is not necessary to the understanding of the autopsy, but is an assurance that the pathologist in training who did the work is completing it in a timely fashion, and the date of transcription assures the world that the typist who must put the dictation on paper is likewise doing her work with reasonable promptness. This would seem a small point, but one of the criteria for the approval of a laboratory by the inspection and accreditation program of the College of American Pathologists is the completion of autopsies within sixty days. In this case, the report was ready for the staff pathologist to review and sign forty-three days after the death. This is fairly good. Many hospitals make the sixty-day deadline with only minutes to spare and others don't even live up to this standard. A few places get the report to the record room only a week after the death, but these risk doing a sloppy, hurried job.

Thoughtful contemplation is the hallmark of good pathology practice. The only exception to this is when the pathologist must make an immediate diagnosis by frozen section while the surgeon is still operating, to assist him in making decisions on how far to carry the operation. There is rarely an emergency in the autopsy side of pathology.

CHAPTER FIVE

THE CAUSE OF DEATH

When a patient dies, the government of whichever well-organized state or nation where the death occurs requires of some responsible person, generally a physician, a statement as to the cause of death. This is required in most areas before the body can be buried or cremated. The information is then entered into the records of vital statistics, the insurance company proceeds with the payment of any claim, and all the other orderly processes which are needed to close out the public interest in the deceased take place.

Unfortunately, government records of vital statistics can be woefully inaccurate and unreliable because the certification of the cause is, all too often, carelessly done. The doctor certifying the cause is often ready to enter a likely but unproven diagnosis, because he does not see the need for accuracy; the patient is dead and can't be brought back, however precise he is in his certificate, and he usually has little interest in the broad picture of government statistics. He runs no risk of censure or punishment for an inaccuracy here; there is no malpractice risk, and only rarely will his certificate be disputed. Even more rarely will his determination be reversed, through exhumation and autopsy of a buried body. In this matter, it can be truly said, "the doctor buries his mistakes." Even if there is to be cremation, and his determination is reviewed by the medical examiner as it must be in cases coming to cremation, only the most super-conscientious of medical examiners will dispute his certificate.

The obvious course to be taken to assure accuracy in

delineating the cause of death, is to have the results of a well-done, carefully recorded autopsy given to the person certifying the death, so a proper certificate can be made out. Only rarely can the precise cause of death not be determined by autopsy, and the statistics resulting from autopsied death certificates can be relied upon to give a true picture of how our citizens are dying. This is not without significance. Patterns of disease can be identified and action taken to correct dangerous situations on the basis of statistical findings. For example, clusters of a particular disease often give a clue as to the possible hidden cause of that particular disease.

One of the most interesting examples of identifying an unusual cluster of disease occurred, not as a result of autopsy, and not through government statistics, but through a private organization. *American Legion Magazine* tries to keep updated necrology information on its members, and it publishes obituaries routinely. Several years ago, a number of legionnaires scattered over a considerable area died, and it was noted that, in each case, the individual had attended a convention at a hotel in Philadelphia. This information, which would not have appeared through official statistics since the victims were from many different localities, led to an investigation and the subsequent discovery of a brand new disease, dubbed legionnaires' disease. Since this discovery, careful work has identified its cause, mode of transmission and other facts, and has given information leading to appropriate treatment and cure. The magazine's obituary policy, in this case, was a lucky break, but autopsies can be similarly useful in identifying other clusters of disease.

Autopsies are done to determine, with as much accuracy as possible, the cause of death of the individual. Death is described in a variety of ways, depending on the person describing it. One common phrase is "ceased to breathe," but others will use "departed this life," implying that there is an afterlife. The Christian Scientist, denying death which he perceives as evil, will say "passed on." The precise medical and legal people who are struggling with the problem of organ transplantation have a difficult time, since a donor organ cannot be removed from a living person, but the organ itself must be "living" when transplanted. To solve this problem, the concept of brain death is emerging. When it is quite apparent, with an electroencephalogram (brain-wave) recording showing that there is a complete absence of any activity of the brain, then we say there is no hope for life in the sense that the individual personality can be restored. The body can still be kept "alive" by artificial means such as respirators, cardiac pacemakers and so on, but there must be a functioning brain for life of the individual to exist. In most areas, when the brain wave is flat, recording only a straight line, it is appropriate and legal to remove all of the life-support machines, and it is at this time that the still-living kidneys or other organs may be removed for transplant. (See chapter fifteen)

Death does not occur all at once. One organ or system of organs may die some time before another. It is a matter of common knowledge that growth of hair may continue for some time beyond the official death. The pathologist is quite familiar with the fact that muscles will contract upon stimulation for several hours after death, for he sees this clearly in cases where the autopsy is performed promptly after death has been pronounced.

I have heard organic chemists claim, quite rightly given the terms in which they function, that life itself is an extraordinarily complex chemical equation in equilibrium, and that death occurs when this chemical equation is unbalanced and the equation goes to completion, one way or another. I don't expect that most readers will get this concept, and really I can't explain it further; the chemists will understand.

The specific things causing death fall into a number of groups, and perhaps it will be of value to consider a few examples. Naturally, I cannot cover all of the multiple causes, but here are a few:

Blood Loss. This is a familiar cause of death by accident, where blood vessels are lacerated and a significant quantity of blood escapes from the body. The amount of blood must be large enough so that the transport of oxygen to, and carbon dioxide from, the tissues is interfered with. The volume of blood in the average-sized adult human is about six liters (twelve or thirteen

U.S. pints); this has been measured a number of ways, from actually extracting every drop of blood available from an executed criminal, to the addition of a known quantity of radioactive material such as radioiodine by injection, and seeing how much it is diluted by the blood volume of the body. Most people know that it is perfectly safe for a normal healthy person to lose a pint of blood; our blood donor system is founded on this, and the volume loss is made up within an hour from other body fluids, though the red blood cell loss takes several weeks to replace. But if a normal person loses two or three pints of blood, then the remaining volume becomes too small to do all the jobs it must do, and shock is the result. Many nonmedical persons do not understand that shock is a fairly precise term when used by doctors, and means a drop in blood pressure from whatever cause: loss of blood, exposure to electric current interfering with heart action, overwhelming toxins within the bloodstream, or even severe physical or emotional stress; I'll deal with each of these and more later in this chapter. The result of shock is the loss of consciousness because there is not enough oxygen reaching the brain via the bloodstream. If the drop in blood pressure continues, then there may be a permanent loss of consciousness which we call death, because the brain can survive a lack of oxygen for only a very few minutes without permanent damage.

If the individual is abnormal, or in an abnormal situation, blood volume problems may come before the loss of two or three pints of blood. For instance, there may be anemia, where the blood contains fewer than the normal number of red blood cells; the hemoglobin of the red blood cells does the actual transportation of oxygen and carbon dioxide. Or the person may live at a high altitude, where less oxygen is available. A common problem is that the individual may be smaller than average, or a child, and cannot tolerate even a pint of blood loss without going into shock, because the total volume of blood in the body is so much smaller.

Pump Failure. The heart is one of the simplest organs of the body, and the most essential. It is a pump and only a pump, which makes the development of an implantable artificial heart, now an experimental procedure, very possibly a standard therapy for the future; external pumps to replace heart actions are widely used today, generally in operations where the natural heart must be stopped. The heart is so essential that one very common cause of death is the heart attack. In this all-too-common disease, part of the heart muscle dies because its own supply of blood is interrupted by a blockage of one or more of the coronary arteries which originate just at the outflow valve of the heart, and circle back to supply the heart muscle. With the death of some of the heart muscle, the ability of the heart to pump a normal amount of blood is reduced, and if the amount of heart muscle which dies from lack of circulation is large enough, shock and death may come quickly.

Another cause of pump failure is arrhythmia. This is an interruption of the steady rhythm of the heart beat, and the many cells of the heart muscle may start contracting at random, rather than all together to do the work that is needed. This particular arrhythmia is called fibrillation, and while atrial fibrillation is not too serious because it involves only the antechamber of the heart, ventricular fibrillation is rapidly fatal, because it involves the main pumping muscle. Everyone who watches television knows that the patient may be kept going in such cases by external cardiac massage, and that arrhythmia may be corrected by electric shock, but the situation in ventricular fibrillation is desperate, and death comes in only a few minutes if the situation is not corrected. Electric shock is a strange thing because it can cause as well as correct ventricular fibrillation, and whoever decided that our system should supply electricity at sixty cycles per second (as is common today), chose the type of alternating current most likely to disturb the action of the human heart.

A less common complication of a heart attack can be the rupture of the heart; in these cases, the heart muscle which has died from lack of blood actually softens and bursts, filling the space around the heart with blood, and destroying its ability to pump because it is squeezed from the outside. This can happen several days after the heart attack, when the dead muscle is softest, but after a few more days, scar tissue cells invade the area to reestablish a firm wall which still cannot pump, but at least it won't burst.

A related problem is pulmonary embolism, the cause of death of the man in chapter four. An embolism is any abnormal material that gets loose and travels in the bloodstream; so there may be an air embolism, an amniotic-fluid embolism, or a tumor embolism to name (but not explain — sorry!) a few. The commonest type of embolism is the result of the clotting of blood (a thrombus) within a blood vessel, and the subsequent travel of this clot in the circulating blood when it breaks loose from where it was formed. Veins are the common site of such clotting, particularly the veins of the legs, and death from this cause happens as a result of inactivity of the legs, as when a patient is allowed to lie without moving in a hospital bed for too long. It has also happened to normal healthy people who have been sitting without moving for a long time, such as on a long airplane ride. In any case, when activity is restored, the leg-vein clot breaks loose and travels with the flow of the blood, through larger and larger veins until it reaches the right side of the heart; then it is pumped out, through progressively smaller arteries of the lung until it reaches an artery of too-small diameter, where it plugs the artery and stays, so that the portion of the lung supplied by that artery dies (a pulmonary infarct). But if the clot is large enough so it plugs a large pulmonary artery, the whole pumping action of the heart may be stopped because there isn't a place for the blood to circulate — hence death occurs, and very rapidly. Few of these cases of massive pulmonary embolism can be saved, even with prompt surgical intervention.

Air embolism can occur when air is forced into the vein in a large enough quantity to spoil the action of the heart valves; the heart chamber fills with froth and the heart can't pump froth. I recall one case I autopsied of a young man who, with too much alcohol aboard, crashed on his motorcycle on a Sunday morning and was pronounced dead at the scene by the local medical examiner, who ordered an autopsy. I found a level of alcohol in the bloodstream which was insufficient to even approach death, although he must have been fully drunk, about 0.18%; drunkenness begins at about 0.10%, and a lethal level is generally 0.40%

or higher. The autopsy revealed no injury which was sufficient to cause death; he had some broken bones, but no laceration of the skin of any significance. But when the heart was opened, I encountered froth, not liquid blood, so the cause of death was air embolism. Now I was faced with a real problem: how did the air get into the bloodstream? I hunted and hunted with no luck until I opened the large intestine, where I found a large laceration with considerable bleeding. What had happened was most unusual; in falling, the unfortunate young man twisted and lacerated his large intestine just in the location where there was a large bubble of intestinal gas, and this was forced through the laceration into the veins, where it traveled to the heart, causing pump failure. In a way, this was not air embolism. It was flatus embolism!

I could go on and on explaining the causes of death from blood loss or from pump failure, but it would take a whole book on this alone. There are many other causes of death to consider.

Toxicity. This common cause of death can be subdivided into chemical poisons and bacterial toxins, and depending on the individual agent, they work in a number of different ways. For instance, cyanide compounds, even in very small amounts, interfere with the ability of individual cells of the body to absorb and use oxygen, so death is quick. But lead, another familiar poison, interferes with the red blood cells, and in sufficient quantity it can actually coagulate the tissue protoplasm. Arsenic is similar, when given in large enough quantities in the form of soluble arsenic salts. More complicated chemical poisons act in other ways; a barbiturate (a favorite drug for suicide) causes death by depressing brain function until the basic control mechanisms of breathing are disrupted. Alcohol in sufficient dosage causes death by similar mechanisms, although in lesser dosage it can cause death by precipitating accidents or by otherwise interfering with the good judgment of the person who consumes it.

Death as a result of bacterial toxicity has decreased from a common cause to a fairly rare one, at least from bacterial toxins alone. Many people die with pneumonia when sick unto death with other causes. Bacteria can enter the body in many ways, by being breathed in, by being present in contaminated food, by injection through the skin, and even by retrograde passage up the urinary apparatus or through the vagina or rectum. Organisms may enter even directly through the ear, the eye, or the pores of the skin, although the skin is generally an excellent defense against disease. In any case, after entering the body, bacteria grow and reproduce, and they produce poisons as a product of their metabolism. These poisons affect the body, especially the brain, and fevers appear. If the infection is massive enough, and the body defenses weak enough, the toxic products can cause death.

Bacteria. And in this category I should include also the viruses, the rickettsia, the mycoplasmas, the fungi, and even the protozoa that can cause death by interfering with the normal body processes: by ulcerating into blood vessels, blocking lymph channels, causing the body's normal defenses to overreact, setting up abscesses in vital organs, and so on. It's not always the toxins that directly cause the trouble. Cholera, for instance, causes death by so irritating the intestines that they respond with an outflow of fluid, and the body dies of dehydration.

I had an old friend who was in graduate school with me, a skilled bacteriologist working for a state health department laboratory. After World War II he was engaged in reestablishing the bacteriology cultures which had been put away for the duration of the war. He developed sinusitis, which in New England is a very common disease, but it got worse and worse. Someone had an idea and studied the problem further, and he found that the sinusitis was actually caused by a bacterium called in those days *Eberthella typhosa* (now it's been renamed *Salmonella typhi*) which is the organism that causes typhoid fever. It has never been known to cause sinusitis before, but about the time the diagnosis was made, the disease ulcerated through the wall of the carotid artery in a location where the bone structure prevented any control of the resulting hemorrhage so he died, and the autopsy confirmed the diagnosis. Typhoid organisms had gotten into the air of the laboratory when the stored cultures were reopened. As far as I know, this is the only case of this kind ever recorded.

Cancer. The cause of death that is most interesting to pathologists, however, is cancer, because there are so many unanswered questions about it, and there is such a great need for progress in treatment. By understanding more about cancer, we all hope that someday there will be a definitive, effective means of preventing and curing it. Today we have surgery, radiation and chemotherapy, and immunotherapy and hormone therapy are showing considerable promise. But the clear cause of cancer is not understood, and if it were, there probably could be really effective treatment, and possibly even a means of prevention. It appears now that the concurrent effect of many factors is necessary to cause cancer, but if research could direct its work against the one absolutely necessary factor for the development of all cancers, it might well find the "magic bullet" that would change the whole picture.

How does cancer cause death? There are a number of mechanisms. First, cancer is a tremendous load on the metabolism of the body that preempts the food substances that the rest of the body needs; this is why the patient with a cancer is so often thin and emaciated. The uncontrolled growth of cancer cells demands a large supply of nutritional requirements, cheating the rest of the individual out of what is needed for continued life. Most people with cancer eat a normal, or even a large amount of food, but the cancer can cause death by just starving the rest of the body due to its insatiable demands.

More commonly, however, cancer causes death not quite as directly. The malignant growth, by its metabolic demands, weakens the body's defenses against a number of diseases. By starving out the immune system, cancer makes the patient more susceptible to a variety of other diseases. Thus it is common for the cancer patient to die of pneumonia or some other infectious process. Depending on the particular location of the tumor, some cancers predispose the body to some specific infection, such as bladder inflammation in prostate cancer, or peritonitis in perforating stomach cancer. Cancer of the lymph nodes may directly interfere with the immunity defenses of the body, since the antibodies against disease are generally manufactured in the lymph nodes.

Another mechanism by which cancer kills is by mechanically interfering with an organ which is necessary for life. Thus a cancer of the bladder may so effectively block the outflow of urine that the kidneys are destroyed by the back pressure which distends the entire urine collecting system and squeezes the kidney cells to death; this is called hydronephrosis, and no one can live long without kidneys. Cancer nodules can settle in the liver and practically replace the normal liver tissue; since the liver is a very complex organ performing many functions necessary for life, death ensues. Cancer can pinch off either the blood vessels, the breathing apparatus of the lungs, or the intestines, and if surgery cannot correct the situation, the patient inevitably dies. Cancer within the brain can increase the pressure within the skull until the spinal cord is squeezed to death at the point where it leaves the skull.

Still another death mechanism of cancer is invasion of blood vessels, with the formation of openings through which blood may escape, with resulting death from blood-loss. Cancers of the stomach and of the intestines are particularly likely to do this.

The one most common characteristic of cancer is its ability to invade surrounding structures, with destruction and replacement of normal tissues and, depending on the location of the cancer and the vital necessity of the tissue invaded, cancer causes death either rapidly or slowly.

When the pathologist performs an autopsy, and examines the samples of the tissues under the microscope, he learns to recognize the signs of disease and to determine just what disease caused the death. It is rare for the well-trained and alert pathologist to be unable to assign a clear, specific cause of death, or to fail to identify all of the contributing factors that made it possible for the principal and underlying disease to reach an irreversible conclusion. Often several separate causes may exist, any one of which would not have immediately led to the fatal conclusion, but together they are lethal indeed. Thus, for example, the autopsy may show an underlying generalized arteriosclerosis, with arteriosclerotic heart disease, and pyelonephritis of the kidney which caused increased blood pressure, followed by failure of the heart to keep up with the blood pressure demands and an outpouring of fluids into the lungs, and finally broncho-pneumonia, which was the coup-de-grâce. Believe me, this is a fairly simple sequence; many cause-of-death determinations are much more complex.

It would be a mistake not to admit that the pathologist can be wrong. Nobody's perfect, and it is not unusual for further investigation to find some detail that the pathologist has misinterpreted. That is why, in the larger hospitals, there are organ review sessions where all the pathology department staff gathers to review each autopsy case. But the pathologist has a better chance, much better indeed, to approach the complete truth than does the surgeon who has a limited ability to look inside, or the internist who has no chance at all. I must confess that this situation leads to an occupational disease of pathologists, the disease of spurious omniscience; since he has no one to check up on him, he comes to believe that he cannot make a mistake. Other people have humility thrust upon them in no uncertain terms, but the pathologist must develop his own humility without assistance.

Once in a long while, the pathologist is confronted with a case on which he can assign no cause of death. This happened to me only once in a long career; a twenty-eight-year-old woman in good health had gone to Florida from her home in Connecticut for a brief visit, and while there, had fallen ill with no localizing or definitive symptoms, just a generalized malaise with headache, fever, aches and pains. At the urging of her friends, she consulted a local faith healer, in whom she had no real confidence. This practitioner told her that she had been placed under a curse, and that she should not leave Florida until the curse had been lifted. She chose to ignore this advice and returned to Connecticut. Within ten days, her complaints became severe, and in spite of hospitalization and vigorous (but nonspecific) treatment, she died. I performed the autopsy, and could find no anatomic cause of death.

It is important for the results of autopsies to be put together so that clusters of causes of death can be used to identify problems which may lead to premature death. In the small hospital, the pathologist can put together in his own head those things which will point to problem areas. If three cases of meningitis appear on his autopsy table within a short time, he would be quite correct in suspecting an epidemic, and in hitting the panic button to alert both the medical community, and the public press. In larger institutions, with a number of different prosectors performing the autopsies, there has to be a mechanism to identify clusters of disease. Whole communities may be involved, and the local health departments are generally very alert to situations which suggest epidemic or public health aspects of disease problems.

The *Journal of the American Medical Association* maintains an obituary section, and attempts to report the death of every deceased physician in the nation. It used to be part of those obituaries to report the cause of death, but recently the journal has given this up, and instituted a policy of occultation of the cause, much the same as the public press does generally. I fail to see why this was done; it was very useful to get an overview of why doctors are dying. It may have been because of the high incidence of suicide, particularly among psychiatrists. But I think it is a serious mistake to withhold information on the cause of death; this is information which might be useful in identifying clusters of a particular disease that then can be prevented from spreading further, or that at least can be publicized so people are aware of their danger.

I had a dear friend, a dedicated physician, who died following an illness with a diagnosis of bone marrow cancer (plasmacytoma, or multiple myeloma), and I was honored to be given the task of writing an obituary for the newspapers. I insisted on including "died of cancer" because his widow wanted the inclusion of the sentence, "He was a devoted member of Alcoholics Anonymous," and I felt, if the cause were not specified, everyone would say, or at least think, that he died from drink or from cirrhosis of the liver, and his many years of splendid service in helping others with their alcohol problems would be tarnished. He was indeed an alcoholic, and kept his disease under splendid control. His autopsy showed that his liver was completely unimpaired, and that he indeed died of cancer of the bone marrow. Disclosure of the cause of death, in many cases, can stop the wagging of tongues, as I hope it may have done in this case.

It would be useful if the news media would report the cause of death in each obituary, unless the family of the deceased objects strongly. For instance, if the deaths from lung cancer were publicly identified, perhaps more progress could be made in getting people to stop smoking. Not that there hasn't been splendid progress already (in spite of the suggestions of the Tobacco Institute to the contrary); smoking is clearly going out of style, except in the less intelligent segment of young women. But if the lung cancer deaths of some famous people such as Edward R. Morrow, Nat King Cole, and Humphrey Bogart — heavy smokers all — were identified as to cause in the news media, the message of the damage done by tobacco might reach some people who otherwise might continue smoking. John Wayne was a hero to many, and it would have served a very useful purpose to point out in clear, unequivocal terms, that he died of lung cancer, almost certainly in consequence of his smoking. Yul Brunner, before he died of lung cancer, became an enthusiastic advocate of the need to stop smoking.

Several years ago, the famous forensic pathologist, Dr. Thomas Noguchi of Los Angeles, was in trouble with the Los Angeles Board of Supervisors; he had been strongly criticized for revealing causes of death of some famous Hollywood personalities. The examples cited were Janis Joplin, William Holden, Natalie Wood, and more recently, John Belushi, and all of these were drug and alcohol related deaths. Now it should be noted that the strongest criticism came to the Board of Supervisors from persons with organized crime connections. Some people have suggested that the attack on Noguchi was motivated by anti-Japanese racism, but I'm inclined to think that it results from a desire of the drug traffic people not to have it pointed out to the public that drugs cause death.

It is now becoming clear that there is such a thing as death from old age, and that we have our maximum life span programmed into our genetic makeup. But many deaths occur before they need to. The more we understand the various conditions which tend to cause death, the better we can formulate the strategies to avoid premature death. We can't avoid death forever, and it is apparent that most of us wouldn't want to. But dying before our time is unfortunate indeed, and autopsies of those who do die early can help us preserve our own lives to their full spans.

CHAPTER SIX

PERMISSION FOR AUTOPSY AND OTHER LEGALISMS

The authorization by which a pathologist is permitted to undertake an autopsy on a particular body is surrounded by a number of legal difficulties. These difficulties vary widely with the part of the world, and the particular culture involved. Even within a fairly homogeneous culture, such as the United States, there is quite a wide variation because of the fragmentation of the nation into many states, each with its own legislature writing the laws and with varying special-interest pressures causing many differences. The influence of funeral directors' organizations vary from area to area, and the strength of the local medical societies causes a variation of the pressures upon the lawmakers. In this chapter, I will discuss some of the general rules involved in obtaining permission for autopsy in the United States and mention some of the variations from these general rules; but all the points of all the applicable statutes and customs cannot be covered because it would take a large volume on this subject alone to give adequate coverage. The reader must realize that he should make further investigation if he is to understand the details in his own state and locality.

Autopsies in those areas where the legal system is based on English common law are generally done only with the permission of the next-of-kin or by order of civil authorities such as medical examiners or district attorneys. That is not to say that common law is the controlling factor; most jurisdictions have modified common law concepts extensively with various statutes, often confused and confusing. But the common law principle which underlies the various rules set down by legislatures is that the body of a deceased person is, in a sense, the property of the next-of-kin. It is not property in the sense that it may be bought and sold, but it is the right of the surviving spouse or other near relatives to possess the body for the purpose of religious rites, for burial, or for other lawful disposal.

However, this limited property right is subject to the prior claim of the state. When there is a legitimate public interest the state, through an officer such as a coroner, medical examiner, or district attorney, may order the disposition of the body — including autopsy and even burial — as is required by the public interest. To restate this without the cumbersome legalisms, if the authorities have a good reason to investigate the death, they may proceed without permission of anyone, and the survivors can do nothing to interfere. I think it is clear that many cases of murder, suicide, or other violent death must be checked out if responsibility is to be determined and the public protected. Just as clearly, it is apparent that infectious disease is a public responsibility if epidemics are to be controlled, and autopsy is often needed in determining the existence of epidemic diseases. A number of other reasons exist which have an appropriate public concern, and these will be dealt with in chapter nine, in reference to the medical-legal autopsy.

Here I am concerned with autopsy permission as generally asked of the next-of-kin. The scenario occurs over and over: the patient expires after several, and sometimes many, days in the hospital, in spite of the earnest work of the doctors, nurses, technicians, and others. The patient's family has been advised of the imminent demise, and was either present or nearby in the hospital waiting room when breathing ceased and the patient was pronounced dead. Now, about fifteen minutes after the death, the attending physician or the house officer comes to the family, and says, "We would like your permission to perform a postmortem examination." He doesn't say autopsy because this is too stark a word. The family of the deceased, if they have read this book, say, "Of course, doctor; we would like to have an autopsy performed." And the permission form is signed.

If the members of the family of the deceased have not read this book, they may say, "I'm sorry, I don't understand. What do you mean?" And at this point, the doctor has the job of explaining. Some do it well, and others succeed only in producing more confusion. I remember one case where the doctor talked for twenty minutes, and the widow finally said that she would have to talk to her children about it. She was an old friend of mine and asked me, instead of her children, what the doctor was talking about. She was utterly confused and quoted a few of his key words like "examination of the body" and "contribution to medical science," so I told her, much to her surprise, that the doctor was asking for autopsy permission. She agreed immediately and the permission was signed. I performed the autopsy; the deceased was also an old friend, and I was pleased to be able to render this final service.

The autopsy permission form is an interesting document, which has evolved over the years, in response to various legal challenges. It generally contains quite standardized wording; indeed, autopsy permission forms are readily available from companies that specialize in marketing hospital forms and record-keeping equipment. It often happens that this standardized form is given to the hospital's lawyer for approval, and he, in order to earn his money, finds that there needs to be a few minor changes of wording. The hospital then prints its own form, using the lawyer's changes and additions.

A fairly typical autopsy permission form is illustrated on the following page.

To this permission form is sometimes added the provision that the autopsy may be used in processes of medical education, and occasionally the form may include the permission to use parts of the body for organ transplant procedures. Some hospitals include a portion of the form to be used when permission is received over the telephone, in which case there is an additional witness to certify that the conversation took place, generally the hospital telephone operator or a nurse. Of course, this telephone

I, ______________________________, ______________________________
Name *Relationship*

of the late ____ of
Deceased

______________________, give permission to the authorities of the Metro-colossal General Hospital to perform an autopsy on his/her body, for the purpose of determining or confirming the cause of death. I give permission for the removal of such organs or parts as may be needed for further study. This permission is subject to the following restrictions or limitations:

____

____

Signed ______________________________ ______________________________
(date)

Address ______________________________

Witness ______________________________ ______________________________

permission certificate applies only in those states that accept permissions given in this manner. Some states accept telegraphic permission, and a copy of the telegrams giving permission is attached to the form, for the hospital record.

As with any legal document, the permission should be signed and dated, with at least one witness signing; often the doctor obtaining the permission (unless he is the doctor who attended the deceased) is witness, but any appropriate person may sign, and occasionally some other family member will do it. In previous years, most states would not recognize a permission as valid unless it was signed after the fact of death of the patient was known to the signer, so the date and hour had to be after the hour of death as certified by the attending physician. Now most jurisdictions will accept a prior permission by the deceased, but if the signer is a surviving next-of-kin, it is generally wise to obtain the signature after the death. This is in case a surviving signer who agreed earlier changes his mind and thinks differently after the fact of death is known.

The blank lines after *limitations* in the form are included in case the permission-giver wishes to write in such restrictions on the extent of the autopsy as fits with his feelings. After discussion with the doctor, he may feel that autopsy of the head is not to his taste, and he may write in (or ask someone to write in), *no head examination* before he signs the permission. Other familiar restrictions are *limited to the abdomen*, or *limited to reopening of previous operative incisions. All organs to be returned to the body for burial* is a severe limitation, for this would eliminate the retention of even the smallest fragments for tissue sampling, but if the words *except small portions for microscopic study* are added, then the very important microscopic part of the autopsy can proceed.

Sometimes the limitation is *limited to abdominal incision*, and this has been construed to give permission for the removal of heart, lungs, and other thoracic structures through the abdominal incision by opening the diaphragm. Such a permission is not clear, and the pathologist would be wise if he examined only the abdominal organs. Incidentally, such a procedure makes the embalmer's job much more difficult; it's easier and neater to embalm a body with all the thoracic and abdominal viscera removed, rather than partial removal. But limitation is clearly a right of the next-of-kin and if exercised, it must be respected, not only legally, but morally and socially as well. I have seen autopsy permissions read *limited to the removal of eyes for Eye Bank donation*, in circumstances where the hospital quite rightly felt that any procedure done on the body of the deceased person is, in a sense, an autopsy.

Occasionally, we hear stories of a hospital stealing the autopsy — a practice unfair to the survivors and legally dangerous to the thief. Perhaps the reader will have heard of the gold nugget trick, where the bereaved spouse is told, quite falsely, that "we had to use a special instrument which had a large piece of gold as one of its parts, and the gold fell off into the body. If we don't do an autopsy and recover this gold, you'll have to be charged for it." There are endless variations on lies such as this, and while they may get signed autopsy permissions, they may also get subsequent signed court judgments against the permission-getter if a smart lawyer gets wind of the trick.

Tales are told also of stealing the autopsy when permission has been refused by removing organs through existing natural openings, so that no incision of the body is made, on the outer surface at least. The problems of removing whole organs through a stretched-open anus are great, and meaningful diagnoses from organs thus obtained are very unlikely, except for answering a few specific questions. But there are pathologists who claim to have done it, and they're taking some risky legal chances. It seems very foolish to jeopardize an entire career in order to obtain a few items of knowledge which could probably be obtained in another autopsy in the near future.

Many jurisdictions hold that any procedure done to a deceased body requires an autopsy permission or a medical examiner's order, especially any procedure which involves invasion of the body through any opening of the skin. Once I was asked by a medical examiner, "Just stick a needle in and get me a tube of blood." I declined because in that state, I needed valid permission or a valid order written by the medical examiner. He didn't want to put it in writing because he knew that his office would then receive a bill from my hospital, and he had already overspent his budget. So he never found out what the deceased's blood alcohol level was.

My brother tells a story from his time as an intern in a large city hospital many years ago. It concerned the case of an unfortunate man who died after a long course of hospitalization during which a number of diagnostic mistakes and therapeutic misadventures had occurred. My brother had to go out to the home of the surviving spouse, who could reasonably be assumed to be distressed by his untimely death and very angry about the way her husband's illness had been handled. My brother talked all around the question of autopsy, which was urgently desired by the doctors. He cited all the hard work that had gone into handling the case, how interesting and important her husband's illness had been to medical education, and on and on for a couple of hours. At last he could delay no longer and asked outright for autopsy permission, expecting furious refusal. Her response was, "Oh doctor, would you? I wanted an autopsy so much and I didn't know how I could ask you!" It isn't always a difficult selling job to get permission.

Autopsy permission-getting is essentially a selling job, and if the permission-getter is a salesman who really believes in his product, most permissions can be obtained. In my internship year, just out of medical school, I believed in the need and usefulness of autopsies almost as much as I do today. The intern is generally the one charged with getting the permission, at least on ward cases (I trained before Medicare practically eliminated the ward or service case), and I accepted my responsibility with enthusiasm. The result was that I obtained permission in ninety-five percent of the cases that were my responsibility, and I was frequently asked by the attending physicians to get permission on their private cases. The percentage of other members of the hospital staff averaged between seventy and seventy-five percent, only because they were unwilling to put out the effort that I did. Many times I took the hospital station wagon out as much as twenty-five miles from the hospital in order to return with a permission.

Some states (fourteen of them) recognize permission for autopsy signed before death, and permission by the dying patient. This makes it easier to get around one objection of the next-of-kin: "He would not have wanted an autopsy." So many family members feel that they know exactly what the deceased wanted, but they rarely do; generally they are expressing only their own prejudices. But the one statement that really defeats the autopsy permission-getter is the claim: "He made me promise I wouldn't permit an autopsy." Otherwise, the person asking the permission can generally argue, "He was a decent person who liked to help other people, and if he could only know what a help an autopsy would be to mankind, he would have wanted it." But the report of a promise not to grant permission really closes out the entire possibility.

What other objections do people generally give as a result of their primitive anti-autopsy bias? The answer to "My religion forbids it" will be dealt with more fully in chapter ten, "Autopsy and Religion", but I want to state here that, while all religions common here in America demand respectful treatment of the dead body and careful maintenance of the rights of the next-of-kin, no religion common in this country has any absolute prohibition of the autopsy procedure. Generally this objection is only an expression of the prejudice of the deceased's survivors, and is not valid except in terms of the survivor's emotional need. Sometimes an appeal to an authority within the survivors' religion can turn this objection around; the priest, minister or rabbi will often support the principle involved in granting an autopsy.

Another objection, and this is what this book strives to correct, is the idea that "We don't want him mutilated or disfigured." One of my primary objects in writing this book is to stress that there is no mutilation or disfigurement in the sense that the objection is given. The autopsy does not preclude the exhibition of the embalmed body, clothed and lying in the casket which is so important to many people in our culture. If the autopsy has been done properly, I challenge anyone to say whether such a body has been autopsied or not, without opening the clothing or lifting the head to examine the back. I speak of this further in chapter eleven, "The Autopsy and the Funeral Director". If by mutilation, the person means any incision of the body, even if concealed, it is clearly appropriate to argue that the procedure is like a surgical operation, done for a purpose and with respect, and if this be mutilation, it should be accepted for all the good it can do.

Another problem is the answer to a request for autopsy permission which says, "Oh, yes, I'd like an autopsy, but I'm afraid of what Aunt Minnie would say." The response to this could be, "Aunt Minnie need never know," but this is not a good idea in most cases. It is better to say, "May I please talk to Aunt Minnie; I think I can convince her." The result of this, most of the time, will be that this second interview will be found to be unnecessary, and the permission will be granted.

There are many other statements which the next-of-kin may use to justify his resistance to the concept of autopsy. The gamut runs from "We don't care what he died of" to "I thought the doctors knew all about his disease, and an autopsy isn't needed." All of these replies need careful answers by the interviewer, answers which will convey sympathy for the loss, understanding of the uncomfortable feelings which are natural when autopsy is considered by the uninitiated, and the fact — undeniable and absolute — that the autopsy can do no harm, and will probably help someone else. It must be made clear that autopsy is not a gory dismemberment of the body, and that the procedure is done carefully and with respect.

One of the saddest objections to autopsy is the totally illogical statement, "He has suffered enough." Surely the person saying this knows that the suffering is over, and that the autopsy can cause no suffering whatsoever. The sad part comes in the realization that the deceased has indeed suffered, and that the only reasonable response is that the patient has been released from his suffering and is now able to help some other person who is suffering too. Families can generally respond to this, and will sign the autopsy permission. Perhaps even sadder is the antisocial attitude of "I don't want to help other people." Apparently little can be done to persuade such people.

The question of who should give autopsy permission can be a difficult one, depending in which particular jurisdiction the permission is sought. I don't believe that there is any area in this country, or perhaps throughout the world, which doesn't recognize the surviving spouse as the appropriate person to approach primarily for autopsy permission. But if there is no surviving spouse, then there is a wide divergence of custom concerning just who is the appropriate person to sign the permission, and the result is quite confusing. This occurs also if the spouse is incompetent. And what is the effect of a legal separation? A divorced spouse has no rights in the matter, but a separated spouse is another question. Every state has its own rules; some states have a rigid order of preference, so that, if there is no widow or widower, the children of the deceased must be approached, then parents, brothers, sisters, grandparents, uncles, aunts, and so on. Other states say merely that the individual, not necessarily a relative, who represents that he is to assume the responsibility for the care and burial of the body, may give the autopsy permission if the hospital authorities feel that he is acting in good faith in his representations and there appears no objection from the available relatives. Some states require that, if the responsibility falls on the children of the deceased (a very frequent situation since many patients are old and widowed at the time of death), then all children of the deceased must sign the permission for autopsy. It is readily seen that this is often a crippling requirement when there is a large family and one or more siblings of the son or daughter at hand may be off anywhere in the world. This problem is solved in many cases by just ignoring the requirement if the relative at hand says that the family will be in agreement. It is very rare for anyone to cause trouble in such a situation, but hospital administrators get very anxious.

One state, Connecticut, has a statute which provides that an autopsy may be performed with no permission required, if forty-eight hours has elapsed since the death and no relative, friend, or other responsible person can be found, in spite of diligent search. Of course, the hospital authorities will be sure that the diligent search is well-documented, with a record of all telephone calls, telegrams, and other attempts to establish contact carefully kept. In many other states, it is legal for the welfare commissioner or other such person to give permission in the absence of relatives when the individual has been a public charge. Many states have unclaimed-body laws which permit the donation of the body to a local medical school for student dissection, and in many such instances the law can be stretched to include autopsy.

The residents of public institutions who die without relatives are frequently turned over for medical school dissection, but there is increasingly a public concern about possible mistreatment in the institution, and frequently the medical examiner is called to certify the death. Often the medical examiner will order autopsy in these cases, if only to protect the institution from accusations of mistreatment of a person in public charge. This is increasingly the method of handling deaths in mental hospitals, and death in jail almost always requires that the medical examiner be called, even if the cause is clear, in order to document the situation and protect the correctional authorities.

The practice has grown up, without apparent legal challenge, of accepting autopsy permission from ecclesiastic authorities in cases of the death of members of religious orders. As far as I know, there is no statutory justification for this, but many times I have performed autopsies on retired priests from a church-operated retirement home, accepting as valid the permission of the Superior of the institution. This was in a state with a large Roman Catholic population, and was apparently utilized only in this faith. I would have hesitated to autopsy an Episcopal priest on permission from his bishop. Perhaps it is the celibacy rule which places, in Roman Catholic eyes if not in statute, the church in the role of the spouse.

What happens when an autopsy is done without valid permission? This is clearly a violation of the quasi-property rights of the next-of-kin, and can be the basis for a suit against the pathologist, the hospital, and others. An autopsy without any signed permission slip is a rare occurrence, but occasionally a valid permission is lacking. This might happen when a surviving spouse was living, unknown to the physician seeking permission, and the permission was obtained from some other relative in a state where there is a rigid succession of the right to give permission. Another difficult situation might occur if the pathologist autopsied the wrong body in a large hospital with several bodies lying in the morgue at the same time.

It is clear everywhere that an autopsy without permission is not the same as a surgical operation without permission; the latter is assault or physical injury, but a deceased body is not legally a person so there can be no assault of physical injury. The action of the next-of-kin would have to be in terms of mental anguish, and a suit on these grounds is likely to be successful since an autopsy without permission is also a criminal act. Mental anguish cases in other circumstances are often unsuccessful because there is no monetary damage done or any provable loss to the complainant, but when it is associated with a clearly criminal act, juries tend to grant damages as a punishment of the defendant.

The state rarely enforces the criminal complaint with more than a suspended sentence, except when there is real malice, which would not apply in cases of the wrong body being autopsied or of the permission being given by the wrong person.

It is the current practice in bringing suit these days to sue everyone with the slightest connection with the case. Thus in an autopsy without valid permission, it is likely that the hospital will be sued as well as the pathologist responsible. The pathology resident who actually did the autopsy is generally sued, along with his chief or supervisor in the larger hospitals, and the attending physician is also likely to be involved, particularly if he made the mistake of getting permission from the wrong person. As in most situations at law today, the results of suits in these cases very widely, with everything from sizable monetary damages to acquittal of the defendant. When monetary damages are assessed the pathologist is in an uneasy situation because some malpractice insurance carriers are beginning to contend that an autopsy without permission is not professional malpractice, but a civil wrong outside the professional field. Up to now however, insurance carriers have defended these cases and paid damages. The hospital's liability is often clear as being administrative negligence, but sometimes the pathologist has been successful in his personal defense by claiming that his autopsy was performed in good faith, that he believed a valid permission was present, and that no monetary or other damage was done to the complainant.

A special case exists when the body of a very recently deceased pregnant woman is opened in the hope of delivering a living baby by Caesarian section. If the opening is not extended beyond the normal incision for a Caesarian section, then the rule of implied consent would normally be applicable. This rule states that it could reasonably be assumed that consent would be granted, and that delay of the procedure in order to obtain consent would cause irreparable harm. So if death occurs during labor, and the husband is not available to give consent, no liability will result if the only procedure is an attempt to save the baby. Of course, the operation is technically an autopsy, since it is the opening of a dead body, but it is not legally an autopsy unless it is extended beyond the procedure necessary to save the baby's life. This situation is rare enough, and is made even more rare by the device of not pronouncing the death of the mother until after the emergency Caesarian has been carried out.

Deaths in the military service constitute a special problem. The permission of the next-of-kin is not required, and the commander or the surgeon of the particular installation or command may, on his own responsibility, determine that the procedure is necessary to determine the true cause of death or to secure information necessary for the completion of military records. Such an autopsy may therefore be ordered without family permission. This procedure applies only when death occurs to those on active military service. Retired or nonmilitary personnel who happen to die in military hospitals are autopsied only with permission of the next-of-kin. The Veterans Administration hospitals, and other federal government institutions, must obtain family permission, just as in any other nongovernmental hospital. Some states, however, permit the hospital authorities to order autopsy on the bodies of deceased patients in mental hospitals, and those states which do not have this provision can do so by merely asking the local medical examiner (who must be called for every mental hospital death anyway) to order the autopsy.

The legal problems which surround the autopsy consist mainly of the matter of legal permission, but I should mention another related legalism, the question of the pronouncement of death. The word *pronouncement* implies that some statement must be made, but no one knows just what words should be used. The *Harvard Medical Alumni Bulletin* of January 1955 has a long and a very amusing account, presented as real and factual, by Dr. Albert E. Hyman who claimed to have solved this problem in his own way. The story, entitled *De Mortem Dictu*, describes how, on his first day as an intern, he was asked to pronounce a patient dead and, not knowing how to do it, he ascertained that the patient was indeed dead, moved to the head of the bed, and stated in a loud voice, "By the virtue of the authority vested in me by the Commonwealth of Massachusetts and in accordance with the rules and regulation of the Health

Department of the City of Boston, I, Dr. Hyman, a duly authorized intern of the Boston City Hospital do hereby and heron officially pronounce this man dead, and in witness thereof I hereby and in the presence of these witnesses set my hand and signature." The effect of this was, it was claimed, to throw the entire ward, and subsequently the entire hospital into an uproar, because such a thing had never been done before, and he was called to the superintendent's office. The upshot of the long story was that the superintendent ordered that, in the future, pronouncement of death would be made in exactly the words he used.

By the time I was around the Boston City Hospital, however, there was no such order in existence, and pronouncement of death was handled in what appears to me to be the most frequently used: the intern, after appropriate tests to make sure that the patient is truly dead (such as listening for heart sounds with his stethoscope, testing for eye reflex and other procedures), goes to the nursing station and takes the patient's chart. He writes "ceased to breathe at 3:10 A.M." or just "pronounced dead at 3:10 A.M." The note is dated and signed, and this appears to cover any legal requirement. He does not need to "pronounce" anything, and he does not, as I did with the first hospital death I had to deal with as an intern, draw up the sheet to cover the face or do any other dramatic act.

The "lawful disposal of the body" is another question to deal with, although it is only peripherally connected with autopsy. The public health laws of the various states have long and specific procedures which must be followed, and while the laws vary from state to state, the general provisions are similar. Following the pronouncement of death the doctor must make out a death certificate, and then the funeral director can assume possession of the body as agent for the family. Transportation of the body must be by a licensed undertaker; removal of the body in the family station wagon is against the law. Generally if transportation is to cross state lines, the body must be embalmed before traveling, but there are many exceptions to this rule.

There are only two legal ways to dispose of a body in the United States, by burial and by cremation. Even if the body is to be given to a medical school, it must be either buried or cremated after the medical school is through with it. Either burial or cremation requires that the local municipality issue a permit, and such a permit cannot be issued until the death certificate has been made out and signed. In most states, the body must be buried in a licensed cemetery. You can't have the burial behind the garage on your own property. And with cremation, the body must be held for forty-eight hours and viewed by the medical examiner (who charges a fee) before cremation, just in case there might appear a need for an autopsy, or in the case of an autopsied body, a re-autopsy for medical-legal purpose.

There is little in the laws relating to the disposal of ashes following cremation, or "cremains," as the funeral directors like to call them, but some jurisdictions require that they be buried or stored in a niche in a licensed cemetery. In most jurisdictions, the scattering of ashes is entirely legal, and the survivors will generally pick a site which is sentimentally connected with the deceased. In California, where cemetery space is becoming quite limited, funeral directors have begun offering a service of scattering the ashes at sea from an aircraft.

The funeral director is in a position to know all the legal requirements relating to the disposal of a dead body, and can be a very valuable protection to the family in making sure that all the legalities are covered. It is unfortunate that some funeral directors will state or imply that some things are legally required when they are not, such as cement vault liners. The family may face certain nonlegal requirements by the gravediggers' union, about which they can do little.

We should not leave this subject of legal problems without mentioning a painful problem with both ethical and legal aspects. Every once in a while, there is a sophomoric individual who utilizes the autopsy as an attention-getting mechanism, and the harm that such a person does is incalculable. I'm speaking of the immature medical student or other person of arrested mentality who obtains an ear or some other part of the body, and uses it to shock people. This seldom happens after the medical school years and, even in medical school, anyone caught doing such a thing should be summarily dismissed as not being good doctor material. What such people risk is not only dismissal but also prosecution, since such handling of body parts is clearly illegal in most states, and the transportation of body parts or the attempt to mail such souvenirs will clearly involve such people in federal charges. But worst of all, such activity displays a total lack of understanding of the serious purpose of anatomical dissection, and a repulsive lack of respect for the body of the deceased. Even the reference to the cadaver as a "stiff" is very rare among medical people, and is found almost exclusively among laymen who wish to demonstrate a spurious aplomb concerning death.

CHAPTER SEVEN

THE HAZARDOUS AUTOPSY

There are few things in human activity which do not have some aspect of danger, and the performance of the autopsy occasionally may have some elements of hazard to the prosector and to those around the autopsy room. It is important therefore that the area where any autopsy is performed be regarded as a contaminated area, and suitable precautions be taken. The elements of deadly disease may be present in any autopsy, and it is impossible to predict which particular case may harbor infection. The wise pathologist regards every autopsy as dangerous, and acts accordingly.

My father, who was a pathologist before he switched to internal medicine (it was easier to switch in the days before the organization of the specialty boards, and most of the best internists had extensive experience in pathology before proceeding to clinical practice) told me a story from the time of his training under the celebrated pathologist at Boston City Hospital, Dr. Frank Burr Mallory, whom I mentioned in chapter two, "The History of Autopsy." The pathology department at the Boston City was charged with providing autopsy service to a number of smaller city hospitals, and one day my father was called to examine the body of a patient deceased at the Mattapan Hospital, then a chronic-disease facility. He took his kit and went to Mattapan, only to find that the diener who made up the kit had neglected to put in rubber gloves. So he proceeded with the autopsy barehanded, ordinarily a completely safe procedure if hands are washed thoroughly afterward. He brought back the tissue samples for processing into slides for the microscope, and in due course, examined the slides and tried to complete the case. There were some puzzling findings, however, so he took the slides and write-up to Dr. Mallory for review. After some study, Dr. Mallory asked my father how long it had been since he performed the autopsy, and on hearing "five weeks," said "That's interesting. You've been dead for three weeks. This is a case of glanders!"

As a matter of fact, Father never showed any of the symptoms of glanders. The disease is a very severe infection caused by a small bacillus called *Malleomyces mallei*, which is endemic among horses and donkeys, and occasionally affects those who work with these animals. It can enter the human body through the intact skin, through the conjunctiva of the eye, by eating contaminated food, or by inhalation. It is extremely pathogenic in the human, and causes severe prostration, fever, chills, nausea, vomiting, and generalized malaise, all of which may come on within a few hours after infection. A pus-filled abscess develops at the site of inoculation, and then multiple abscesses develop along the lymph channels which drain the area of primary infection, followed by abscesses in the liver, spleen, lungs, and muscles, with meningitis frequently a consequence. Death occurs in a couple of weeks in eighty to ninety percent of persons infected, and the remainder will live with chronic glanders, a disease of multiple skin abscesses and low-grade fever, for a few months or years. Half of those with chronic glanders die of the disease eventually.

Some cases of glanders respond to treatment with streptomycin, tetracycline, and chloramphenicol, but my father performed the autopsy thirty or more years before these drugs were discovered. It was just luck that he never developed the disease, and without that luck I wouldn't be here to write this, because this occurred in 1912 and I was born in 1915. It is dangerous enough to autopsy a case of glanders with rubber gloves and other protection, but to do a full postmortem barehanded is extraordinarily hazardous.

Glanders is fairly rare in America, but more common in Asia. It is not often a problem for the American pathologist. Its cousin, anthrax, is somewhat more common here, but the real hazards of autopsy in this country are tuberculosis and infectious hepatitis, and in recent years, AIDS. The entire spectrum of infectious disease has been implicated at one time or another as a cause of autopsy room infection, but tuberculosis leads all the rest with infectious hepatitis a close second.

My own personal experience with tuberculosis is to the point. In 1968, I went for a short period of service at the Hôpital Albert Schweitzer in Deschapelles, Haiti. This splendid hospital, built and administered by Dr. and Mrs. W. Larimer Mellon, serves a very large population of indigent rural Haitians in which the predominant health problems were tuberculosis, tetanus, and malnutrition. In addition to my principal task of improving the arrangements in the clinical laboratory of the hospital, I had the opportunity to autopsy a number of deaths from tuberculosis, and deaths from other causes in persons with tuberculosis. Since I knew of the diagnosis of tuberculosis in these cases, I took more than the usual precautions. I wore double operating gowns, rather than the usual apron over my scrub suit. I wore cap and double mask, which I usually do not do, and I wore two pairs of rubber gloves, one over the other. The cases were interesting and instructive, and were very different from the usual cases I had seen in the Boston area. But the point of this story is: three months later I had tuberculosis, and I heard later that the diener who assisted me on the autopsies also developed the disease. I had the onset of fever, cough, and weakness, and X-ray showed a wedge of infiltrate in my left lung. Gastric washings were obtained, and six weeks later (it takes that long to grow the tubercle bacillus in a test tube) it was reported that these were positive for tuberculosis. My doctor had prescribed erythromycin for pneumonitis, and my fever had disappeared, but I now started on eighteen months of isoniazid hydrochloride and para-aminosal-icylic acid, which are highly specific to cure the disease. I never had to be hospitalized, and I was absent from work only one week — and that was before the diagnosis was made.

I was lucky to have tuberculosis when INH and PAS (that's how the two medicines I took are referred to) were available and effective. Only a few years before, I would have been sent to a sanatorium for a minimum of six months. And today, the tuberculosis bacteria have become resistant to those medications, the incidence of tuberculosis is rising, and treatment is becoming more difficult. Anyway, in spite of all my careful precautions, I became the victim of what I must assume was an autopsy room infection. Historically, tuberculosis was the "pathologist's disease", and many old-time pathologists had it. Even today, many pathologists decline to perform an autopsy on a known tuberculosis death, feeling that the information to be gained does not justify the risk.

The hazard of infectious hepatitis is now perhaps even more significant than tuberculosis, since there is a specific treatment against the tubercle bacillus, but the hepatitis virus has no really good treatment and the long-term problems of liver damage are so very great, with postnecrotic cirrhosis causing death in a number of cases. Hepatitis occurs in two forms, the type which enters the body through the mouth from contaminated food or water (or rarely through the respiratory tract), and the type which is carried into the body with infected needles, lancets or scalpels, or is introduced directly into the bloodstream by infected blood transfusions or serums. The first type, called hepatitis A, takes only three to six weeks to develop, but the second, hepatitis B, is often delayed for between three to five months before it produces symptoms.

Obviously, the greatest autopsy room danger is from the hepatitis B, or homologous serum-type of hepatitis. I would hate to have to estimate the number of times I have nicked myself with a scalpel, or torn my glove and skin on a spicule of bone in the course of an autopsy. Most surgeons will testify that they also often penetrate their own skin in the course of an operation, and while hepatitis is not present in every person, there are a large number of individuals who harbor the hepatitis virus as carriers. The danger of infection from random exposure to blood of another person is very real.

I recall the case of a surgeon who operated on a case of abdominal pain and jaundice, expecting to find a diseased gall-bladder, but found instead a swollen, acutely inflamed liver from hepatitis. He cut himself in the course of the operation, and three months later he developed hepatitis. The patient had died shortly after the operation, and then the surgeon himself died of hepatitis. The surgeon's body was autopsied, and the pathologist, the chief of the department, had the bad luck to cut himself during the autopsy! However, the pathologist survived and indeed showed no symptoms of the disease that had already killed two men. The apparent reason for his survival could be attributed to the fact that he was given injections of gamma globulin, but I believe that it was more due to the fact that he was not a habitual alcoholic. The first patient who was operated on was a known alcoholic, and the surgeon, although no one had attached the alcoholic label to him, was a heavy user of alcohol. Hepatitis is always worse in the alcoholic. Apparently, liver cells that are not exposed to alcohol are much more able to resist the hepatitis virus.

The disease which is probably the most frightening to the pathologist today is Acquired Immune Deficiency Syndrome, familiar to everyone as AIDS. This disease is most alarming because there has been no effective treatment worked out as of the time of this writing. I sincerely hope that by the time this book reaches the reader, an effective therapy will have been discovered which will make the disease no longer the horror it is today. It is a horror because it is so inexorably progressive, and only a death of wasting and deterioration can be seen by the patient when the diagnosis is made.

This does not mean that every person who is infected with the AIDS virus, known as the human immunodeficiency virus (HIV), will inevitably develop the disease. It now appears that some people may harbor the virus for years, and live to infect other people. But many authorities suspect that most of those who are infected will eventually succumb to the full-blown disease, unless effective treatment can be found; it's only a matter of time.

Of course, no one dies directly of HIV infection. The problem comes from the fact that HIV destroys the ability of the body to resist diseases, by spoiling the immune system, which is the most important defense we have against a number of diseases. Thus the AIDS patient may die of infection by *Pneumocystis carinii*, a common organism which otherwise rarely gives any trouble because the immune system is so effective against it. Another disease which can kill the patient with AIDS is Kaposi's sarcoma, a disease that appears as a malignant tumor of the blood vessels of the skin, and which was very rare until the AIDS epidemic. Kaposi's sarcoma was originally described by a doctor whose name was Cohen; he came from the town of Kapos in Hungary, and so he adopted the name Kaposi, because there were already six dermatologists in Budapest named Cohen.

The pathologist must be conscious of the risk of AIDS infection, although I know of no documented case of a pathologist becoming infected at the autopsy table. However, because the disease is so lethal, the pathologist must take particular precautions when autopsying a case of AIDS — and the infection has now become so widespread that every body on the autopsy table should be handled as it were a proven case of AIDS. But the precautions are no different from those necessary for prevention of infectious hepatitis, which is a closely related viral disease.

One of the great scourges of history has been syphilis, so it is the obvious question to ask if this disease is a danger to the prosector during the autopsy. Surprisingly, the risk is quite low. The reason is that the syphilis organism enters the body through the mucous membranes and not ordinarily through the skin, so it would require a splash of infected material into the mouth or the eye, or possibly infection could be introduced through a wound of the skin. Another factor that makes syphilis less of a hazard is the extreme sensitivity of the organism, *Treponema pallidum*, to changes in temperature and to drying. The bacterium dies if its environment drops significantly below body temperature for even one minute, so infection would have to occur by direct transfer of uncooled infected material, and most autopsies are performed on bodies that have lain in the hospital's refrigerator for some time. Drying inactivates the organism in blood or other infected material on the instruments and autopsy table surfaces, whereas in the case of tuberculosis or infectious hepatitis and many other diseases, such material remains hazardous for a long time.

A related problem, really a side issue from the autopsy, but mentioned here to help with an understanding of syphilis, is the question of transmission of the disease in blood transfusion. Most people who have served as blood donors know that one reason for rejecting a potential donation of blood is a history of syphilis. And yet, practically all blood used for transfusion is stored in a refrigerator for some time before it is given to a patient. The syphilis organism is unequivocally dead under these circumstances, so why is the donor rejected? Apparently, it is a survival from the old days of direct transfusion, pumping blood directly from the donor's vein to that of the recipient, and under these circumstances syphilis was a very real hazard, since the blood never cooled. Perhaps there is also a feeling that the potential donor with syphilis is an "unclean person," and has probably led a life that makes it likely that he has other diseases which are transmissible in banked blood. Mostly however, it is simply an unscientific prejudice against the syphilitic donor, and I would not hesitate to use banked blood from a syphilitic donor with no other health problems as a safe transfusion for a patient, especially in any emergency situation.

I should also say that it is very uncommon to pass on syphilis infection from any individual who has had the disease for more than two years, by any means whatsoever. In view of this, the patient who dies of syphilis is no hazard to the pathologist, but only the patient who dies of another disease who happens to have a recent infection of syphilis. Syphilis is such a slow-moving disease that death from syphilis generally occurs many years after the primary infection. The spirochete of syphilis is an organism which has almost learned to live in harmony with the human, but not quite yet. All in all, syphilis, for all the fear and emotion with which it is surrounded, is not a great hazard in the autopsy situation.

The other bacterial diseases should all be considered in any discussion of autopsy room infection, and it is manifestly impossible to undertake a complete discussion of the entire range of these diseases here. Perhaps the more common infections are the staphylococcus, streptococcus, meningococcus and pneumococcus diseases. The latter three are easily treated with penicillin or other antibiotics and so are not a great problem, but staph can cause either boils and other local lesions, or bronchopneumonia, intestinal inflammations, sinusitis, and osteomyelitis. Though it can be very difficult to treat, it lacks the spreading invasiveness of the other coccus diseases and is not commonly any great problem to the individual who is in otherwise good health. Ordinary care in the performance of an autopsy can prevent any problem with these diseases; and likewise, typhoid fever and related intestinal diseases rarely cause autopsy room infection, since the require actual ingestion of infected material except under very special circumstances. I told in chapter five of my friend who died of airborne typhoid which manifested itself as an eroding sinusitis that eventually penetrated the carotid artery and caused him bleed to death, but this was a laboratory infection and not an autopsy room problem.

The protozoan diseases — amebiasis, malaria, leishmaniasis, and trypanosomiasis — are hazards which ordinary care should effectively prevent. Indeed, it would require a conscious effort to infect the prosector in the autopsy situation, and carelessness alone would probably not be sufficient. Not so the fungus diseases, especially histoplasma, coccidioides, and candida. The response of the individual to these infections varies widely, and while they are all highly infectious, many people appear to be able to handle infected material and never develop the diseases they cause. The intestinal tract is not the method of contracting fungal diseases that concerns the autopsy room — it is not a likely route. But airborne infection can occur, and wound infection is a real problem. Candida may infect skin surfaces, but its preferred locations, such as the axilla and groin, are generally not explored during the autopsy. The rickettsial diseases — typhus (different from typhoid fever), Rocky Mountain spotted fever, tsutsugamushi disease, and others — all require transmission by ticks or insects, and so are no hazard whatsoever in the autopsy room.

Viral diseases are a very real hazard. I have already spoken of infectious hepatitis and human immunodeficiency virus, but there are a number of others which can cause problems, Thus herpes virus, psittacosis and several others have been implicated, but again, normal precautions should be sufficient to protect against these diseases. Some of the arboviruses, such as yellow fever, require an arthropod (like the mosquito) for their transmission and can be disregarded. Smallpox has disappeared from the scene, but even in previous years the vaccinated pathologist could safely handle a smallpox case. Today the problem for the pathologist appears to be in the group of diseases called slow viruses, which may produce disease even years after infection. This whole group of diseases, with strange names like Creutzfeldt-Jakob disease, is currently under investigation and is poorly understood. Probably they are not viral diseases at all; it appears that they are caused by agents called mycoplasma that are extremely hard to kill and which result in a number of central nervous system diseases. Hopefully, by the time this book is published, a great deal more will be known about the slow viruses, but right now, they are so poorly understood that it is difficult to begin to estimate how much of a hazard they are to the pathologist. There has never been a proven case of autopsy room infection in this group, but the pathologists continue to worry and to avoid possible exposure.

All in all, there are many infectious disease hazards to the prosector and others in the autopsy room, and I have been able to speak of only a few. However, I can say that most of them, and probably all of them, are preventable by ordinary precautions and careful work, and that the well-trained prosector should be able to do an autopsy safely on any dead body, no matter what the cause of death. Autopsy room infection has to be the result of a break in technique, and I have often tried to reconstruct what break in technique allowed the tubercle bacillus to enter my lungs in the Albert Schweitzer Hospital; perhaps indeed, my infection was acquired on the street, in a bus, or somewhere not related to my performance of autopsies at all, but still the autopsy room seems the most likely.

Other autopsy room dangers exist in the field of accident. In former days, when a rotating electric saw was used to cut bone, there were occasional lacerations and even the loss of a finger when the saw slipped. But the use of the oscillating saw has almost completely removed this hazard. The use of sharp blades is always dangerous, and scalpels and long knives are essential for the work, but most of the other instruments are innocuous. The most common autopsy room injury is a strained back from lifting the body onto or off the autopsy table, but this can be prevented by keeping the back straight when lifting, or by the use of mechanical hoists to move the body.

One more danger to the prosector remains to be spoken of: the hazard in the autopsy of a radioactive body. This does not mean the body of someone who has died in an accident involving radioactivity; the likelihood of exposure of the pathologist and diener to damaging radiation in this situation is so small as to be negligible. I am speaking here of the autopsy of the body of a patient who has been treated with radioactive medications. In recent years radioactive treatment for malignant disease has increased, so the prosector may be confronted with the possibility of a significantly high dosage of ionizing radiation coming from the body itself. Radiation safety standards have been developed which should protect the workers in the autopsy room, but it should also be remembered that there is no safe level of radiation exposure, only a level under which significant damage is less likely to occur. The standards in effect only try to keep exposure to a low level.

Radioisotopes used in the treatment of malignant disease include mostly radioactive iodine (I^{131}) used in thyroid disease, radioactive gold (Au^{198}) used for the treatment of fluid collections in the abdomen or chest and for cancer of the prostate, and radioactive phosphorus (P^{32}) used against leukemia. In the amounts used, these can be a significant hazard to the pathologist if death and autopsy follow soon after the patient has been treated with the radioactive material. If death occurs some time after treatment, the hazard disappears because radioactive gold, for instance, gives up its radiation at the rate of twenty-six percent each day, so that after several days the amount of radiation becomes negligible, though it never completely disappears. The twenty-six percent reduction occurs in the remainder each day in a series such as this: seventy-four percent remains after one day, fifty-five percent after two days, forty percent after three days, and so on down to two percent at the end of thirteen days. It is clear then, that by two weeks after treatment, the body can be regarded as practically nonhazardous. The decay of radioactivity is somewhat slower in radioactive iodine, and slower still with radiophosphorus, but in any case, if the medication has been administered some time before, it is relatively safe to proceed with the autopsy.

If death occurs soon after radioactive treatment and autopsy permission is obtained, it may be possible to delay the autopsy and store the body in the morgue refrigerator, waiting for the radioactivity to cool down to safe levels. But if social pressure or scientific interest dictate the need for an autopsy sooner, there are a number of steps which may make the autopsy safer. Generally, a radiation safety officer (and every hospital should have one) should be consulted, and if his measurement shows less than five millicuries of activity the autopsy may proceed in the usual manner. If the reading is higher than five millicuries, the precautions taken should include the use of heavy rubber gloves to protect the hands, long-handled instruments to manipulate the organs, and prompt removal and segregation of the particular organ where radioactivity is concentrated, such as the thyroid treated with radioactive iodine, or the kidneys treated with radioactive gold; these organs may be refrigerated or placed in formalin fixative for later dissection when the radioactivity has cooled down.

With a very radioactive body it is possible to use a team approach, with two or more prosectors in succession performing the autopsy, so that no one person gets a heavy dose of radiation. The maximum exposure standards are not more than 0.3 R per week to the hands, and not more than 1.5 R per week to the whole body; the radiation safety officer can monitor these figures.

Two special precautions should be observed in the face of radioactivity: special care must be taken to avoid contamination of the autopsy room for obvious reasons, and the funeral director must be informed of the hazard so he can take appropriate precautions. This also applies in cases of infectious diseases as well; the funeral director and his embalmer have a right to be protected.

There are some real hazards to the pathologist and his staff in the performance of some autopsies, but these cases are not frequent, and when they occur the procedure can be done safely if some fairly simple precautions are observed.

CHAPTER EIGHT

THE SPECIAL TOOLS OF THE AUTOPSY
THE MICROSCOPE AND THE MICROTOME

Two very special tools are required for the successful completion of the autopsy. The microscope is essential for the study of the tissues taken at autopsy, and the microtome is essential for the preparation of those tissues so that they can be seen through the microscope. The microtome is used only in the preparation of the histologic slides and is hence limited to the field of pathology. The microscope has applications in other fields, but is so essential in pathology that it deserves special consideration.

THE MICROSCOPE

The microscope is a study itself, with a fascinating history, and with many complexities which result from the physical laws of optics. The precise controls and the fine lenses make this instrument a real engineering triumph, and also a very expensive piece of equipment. It is not unusual for a pathologist to order, for his own use, a microscope costing from three to five thousand dollars. He is generally more economical with the microscopes he buys for his technicians, but even there, a thousand dollars is not unusual.

Many microscopes are made in many forms for various special problems — metallurgy, microdissection, legal ballistics, and so on. The microscope used by the pathologist is one that magnifies an object that is lighted by transmitted, rather than reflected, light; the object is generally a thin slice of tissue mounted on a glass slide and stained with various dyes. In a typical arrangement, the object is placed on the stage of the instrument, and a bright light is reflected by a mirror through a complex lens system (the condenser) to illuminate the object from below. (There are many variations.) The image from the illuminated tissue is brought into focus by an even more complex series of lenses — a lower group called the objective and an upper group called the ocular — so that the microscopist sees the image greatly enlarged in a circular field which appears to be eight or ten inches below the eyepiece. The enlargement may vary from 35× to as much as 1500×, depending on the combination of lenses used. Usually the microscope is provided with a nosepiece on which three, four, or five different objectives are mounted, so a flick of a finger is all that is needed to change from one magnification to another.

Most pathologists, except those who are blind in one eye, prefer to use a binocular microscope, which introduces the problem of separating the image into two oculars by prisms and mirrors, so that two eyes may see the same picture at once. It's not really necessary to see the same picture with both eyes, but the pathologist who must spend hours at the microscope generally finds it more restful to use a binocular instrument. The skilled microscopist who is trained to use a monocular instrument has to learn to ignore the image seen by the eye which is not looking into the microscope, because to shut the eye results in great fatigue. Indeed, those who learn to sketch the object seen will often use the monocular microscope with the left eye, and have the sketch paper under the right eye, so that it is unnecessary to move the head at all, but just to "turn on" the mind's attention first to one eye and than to the other.

The word *microscope* was apparently first used in the Academia Dei Lincei in Italy in 1624; Galileo is said to be the first scientist to use the instrument. A quarter of a century before, the first compound (that is, having more than one lens) microscope had been made by Hans and Zacharias Janssen in Middelburg, Holland. By 1662, the sliding tube whereby the early microscopes were focused was replaced by a screw which gave much more accurate control.

The lens system of these early days were of limited usefulness because the lens grinding was so inaccurate. The next step was then, in a sense, a step backward, because the next significant development in microscopy was the discovery by Anton van Leeuwenhoek that a single lens of extremely short focal length, ground with real precision, could give even better magnification than the compound microscopes then in use. He became quite famous for his microscopes and personally manufactured several hundred instruments, some on commission from the crowned heads of Europe who were fascinated by the new scientific instrument. The precision of these devices was great enough that van Leeuwenhoek was able to demonstrate protozoa and some of the larger bacteria. His instrument utilized a spherical lens which, if held very close to the eye, gave a really greatly enlarged image. The interesting characteristic of the spherical lens is that the smaller the sphere, the greater the magnification and the closer it must be held to the eye. Many early scientists declined to use the microscope because it was uncomfortable to hold it so close. But it produced an acceptable image, at least in the central portion of the lens; the edges had great distortion of the image.

An interesting variant of van Leeuwenhoek's microscope was Gray's instrument of 1696, which used as a lens a tiny drop of water, small enough so it remained essentially a sphere because of the surface tension. Larger spheres distorted considerably with gravity, but a tiny drop was quite successful.

The first anatomist of real stature who used the microscope was Marcello Malpighi, mentioned in chapter two. He worked in the fields of zoology and botany as well as human anatomy, and his pioneering work on the embryology of the chick was a classic of scientific discovery. Many of his accomplishments depended on his use of the microscope. In human anatomy his description of the nature of the liver, the spleen, and the kidneys was classic. He was known as a gentle, sensitive physician and an accurate scientific observer who suffered bitter attacks of jealous colleagues.

Following Malpighi, microscopes improved in consequence of better lens grinding, and the compound microscope became firmly established. Various problems with the earlier instruments were solved, and the power of magnification was steadily increased. Special improvements in the shape of lenses reduced spherical aberration (that characteristic which produced an image in good focus only at the center of the field of vision), but this problem continued for many years and has only recently been fully solved. Another problem was the fact that a lens handles light of different wavelengths differently; violet light is bent by the lens more than red light, so the image produced would be in good focus in only one color, with the other colors out of focus. This was improved with the achromatic lens, and solved with the apochromatic type, using a doubled or tripled lens made up of glass of several different densities. These are called crown glass, flint glass, and fluorite glass, and by combining them in various ways it has been possible to make all colors focus at the same level.

The control of focus was improved by the use of very fine screws or cams, making it possible to produce an image quickly and keep it in focus. The use of metal (first brass and later steel) replaced the ivory, bone and other materials which had earlier been used, and which were subject to wear and distortion.

An interesting development came fairly early in microscope construction. It was always a problem to illuminate the object being examined. Candle flames or other sources of artificial light proved unsatisfactory because the light played on a tiny object had to be spread out over a large area in making the image so it became quite dim. Obviously, the best illumination was the sun itself, and this was so brilliant that it was soon found that the microscope could be used as a microprojector, spreading the image on a large screen in a darkened room As early as 1744, such devices were in use. The sun had remained the best microscope illuminator until very recently. Really satisfactory microscope lights have been in general use only during the past forty or fifty years. But very early on, projected images using sunlight were a common feature not only of scientific gatherings, but also of social events. Carbon arc lights made it possible to project images of microscopic material at night in the early twentieth century, and these are generally replaced today by very high-intensity incandescent light bulbs.

Magnification reached a limit of about 500× enlargement, which was insufficient for really fine details, but then it was discovered that by placing a fluid between the object being examined and the lens system, greater magnification could be obtained. At first water was used, but then oils with about the same refractive index as glass itself made even greater magnification possible. Even greater resolving power was achieved by using shorter wavelengths of light at the violet end of the spectrum and even invisible ultraviolet light was used, with a fluorescent screen to allow viewing. This latter procedure proved cumbersome, and has been superseded by the electron microscope which is explained later.

By the year 1880 or thereabouts, the microscope had reached the basic design of today, and had reached the limit of its power to produce an enlarged image. For very good reasons known to the scientist of optics, no detail smaller than a half-wavelength of light can be defined by the microscope. This is why ultraviolet light, with its shorter wavelength, was tried as an agent for getting a little more magnification. But for general use, the microscope had reached the end of its power to magnify. Many improvements have been made, such as nonreflective coating of lenses, binocular viewing tubes, the addition of the mechanical stage whereby the object being examined can be moved about under the lens with precision, but from the point of view of the physics of optics, the ultimate light-microscope has been with us for more than a hundred years.

Many special devices have been found to improve the usefulness of the microscope, such as dark field illumination, in which the light is brought in from the sides, so that the object is brightly lighted, but no other light except that reflected from the object passes up the tube to the eye. This is essential in identifying the syphilis organism *Treponema pallidum*, which cannot be stained and examined by transmitted light. Polarizing screens permit the identification of many crystal substances, not just in metallurgy, but in human anatomy where the diagnosis of silicosis and similar diseases caused by foreign crystalline materials may be made by polarized light. Phase microscopy has been added. This depends on the interference of two beams of light to make some refractile materials stand out in brilliant detail without staining.

The common pathologist's microscope of today is an instrument with a heavy U-shaped base, and sturdy frame supporting a four-inch square of metal, called the stage, with a central hole. Light reflected by a mirror, or from a built-in illuminator, passes through a series of lenses (the condenser) up through the hole in the stage to illuminate the glass slide or other object passed over the hole. Above this is the viewing tube, with the objective lenses just above the specimen. Generally there are three, four, or even five objective lenses which can be rotated into position, with magnifications of 2½×, 10×, 20×, 45×, and 95× or 100× available with a flick of the fingers. The 95×–100× objective is used with immersion oil. Above the rotating nose-piece on which these objective lenses are installed, the light passes up a tube to the ocular lenses, just 16 centimeters above the specimen. Or today, more commonly, the light path is split by prisms to pass up two tubes to two oculars, set so that two eyes may view the same field at once. The oculars are basically two lenses (but each with several parts to correct for various wavelengths of light) having a magnifying power of 10×–15× enlargement. The result is that the microscopist has at his fingertips magnification ranging from 25× (the 2.5× objective plus the 10× ocular) to 1500×, using the 100× objective and 15× oculars. This whole apparatus is focused by a large wheel, the coarse adjustment, and a small wheel, the fine adjustment, on either side of the instrument.

While the light-microscope is the basic instrument of the pathologist's work area, neither pathologists nor other scientists who work with microscopes were satisfied with the wavelength of light limitation of its resolving power. Of course, the micro-scope is the pathologist's dearest possession, the instrument whereby most of his work can be done. My own microscope was given me at age twenty-one by my father, and fifty-five years later, it is still the instrument I prefer to use, over the fancy research-type machines that are popular today. It does not have the inclined binocular head that is common today, so I just incline the whole instrument to use it. But its optics are better than many microscopes available today, and I'll never part with it. Even so, along with other pathologists, I can't help wondering, "What is the nature of the structures that are smaller than can be seen with our light-microscopes?"

The answer is found in the electron microscope. This instrument has now assumed a place beyond being the scientific curiosity it was regarded as all too often in recent years. The problem of getting the resolving power beyond the half-wavelength of light has been solved by using, instead of a beam of light, a beam of electrons generated by a cathode in a manner similar to the familiar TV tube. But while the electron beam of the TV tube is swept across the screen making the many lines which form the picture, the beam of the electron microscope is held steady and focused, using magnets instead of lenses. A magnet can bend an electron beam, just as a glass lens can bend the light beam. The result is that the researcher is no longer limited by the half-wavelength of light, and many fine details are revealed which have increasing usefulness in the study of disease. The image formed by the electron microscope is generally recorded on photographic papers for later study because the electron beam cannot be played directly into the human eye; although it can be visualized by focusing it on a fluorescent screen, most electron-microscope results are obtained by the study of the photographs produced.

With the release from the limitation of the half-wavelength of light, tremendous enlargement of objects can now be obtained. Magnifications in the order of 2,000,000× are commonplace, and I will not state any maximum, since every month brings further improvements. The light-microscope allowed researchers to see some internal structures of the living cell, such as the mitochondria and the Golgi apparatus, but only as tiny structures too small to be examined by this tool; with the electron microscope (called in the laboratory the EM much in the same way as we speak of the TV), the details of these tiny structures are readily seen, and changes within them can be correlated with the various diseases which affect them. Cell membranes used to be seen as fine, indistinct filaments, but with the EM they are seen to be complex structures with significant anatomy and specific variations induced by known diseases. New diseases and new understandings of old familiar conditions have been identified. Until today, the pathologist has been able to do acceptable work with the light-microscope alone, but from now on, no pathologist can regard himself as a completely adequate diagnostician unless he has access to an electron microscope, and can interpret with accuracy the details which may be visualized with the electron microscope.

There is another aspect of the microscope not yet discussed, the practice of photomicrography. A microphotograph is a very tiny picture, but a photomicrograph is a picture of a very tiny object, enlarged so that it may be examined. Many of today's microscopes are made so a camera can be mounted and pictures made of the things seen through the microscope. In previous years, artists were employed to draw the details which the microscopist sees, and in many ways, the picture resulting is more informative, but today cameras are very widely used to make the pictures used in publications and the slides which are projected at educational meetings. Since pathology is so dependent upon the actual appearance of structures, it is easily seen that the presentation of the findings of pathology is dependent upon the presentation of pictures, and therefore the camera is essential, or a very good artist, and these are very rare.

THE MICROTOME

One more instrument which is essential to the practice of pathology remains to be discussed. This is the microtome. Of course, the meaning of *micro-* is small, and *-tome* comes from the Greek for cut. This small-cut device is the essential instrument for the preparation of slides of tissues to be examined under the microscope. I mentioned the use of this device in chapter three, but it has a history nearly as long as the microscope.

The name *microtome* was first used by Jean-Gabril Chevlier

in 1839; prior to this time, they were known as "cutting engines" in English, and something similar in other languages. Johannes E. Purkinje gets the credit as the first pathologist to use the microtome in his work, probably about 1830, and his name is attached to the nerve cells of the cerebellar part of the brain and to specialized fibers in the heart muscle, as a result of his extensive and valuable work. The microtome used in his day was a simple device whereby a hand-held knife could cut a very thin slice of the tissue to be examined, as it was raised by a screw device between two bars on which the knife rested.

Various primitive microtomes were tried, but by 1870, the basic instrument which is still used today was described by Wilhelm His. He described the sliding microtome, whereby a very sharp knife is held to a metal block, which slides along oiled tracks, to cut slices off a tissue raised on a screw-controlled base. Similar instruments had been known for seventy years, but lacked the features which allowed precise control.

The sliding microtome is used today, especially for very large blocks of tissue, such as a whole uterus or even a whole brain. A similar variation, the swinging microtome, is often used for the frozen-section microtome, with carbon-dioxide snow (dry ice) to freeze the tissue, instead of taking the time to process the tissue through the many steps that lead to paraffin embedding and sectioning as I described in chapter three. Freezing hardens the tissue so that it may be cut into fairly good sections, but not as thin as the sections which are obtained with paraffin embedding. The frozen section technique permits the rendering of a diagnosis within a very few minutes after the tissue reaches the pathologist, and is used to advise the surgeon of the nature of the disease while the operation is still going on. The question "Is it cancer?" can be answered, and the answer determines just how much operation the surgeon should do. But the frozen section is not as precise as the paraffin section, and should always be confirmed by a permanent paraffin mount; it is used just for such situations where an answer is urgently needed to control a choice of treatment.

My father, who was a pathologist before he left the field to practice internal medicine (I've mentioned before that most of the best internists of his day were trained pathologists) had a microtome of the frozen section type, which he purchased in 1913. This was the Spencer 821, and the same microtome is made and sold today. The parts of his microtome are interchangeable with today's models.

In 1883, Pfeiffer at Johns Hopkins and Minot at Harvard devised, independently of each other, the rotary microtome. Here the tissue block is held in the jaws of a vise, which moves down against a fixed blade. By this arrangement, the sections cut off the paraffin-embedded tissue stick together, edge to edge, to form a delicate ribbon which can be mounted on a glass slide. The Minot type of microtome is still very popular today, but even more popular is the Spencer 820 which is such a perfect machine that no one has found a way to improve it in fifty years or more, beyond giving it a fancy case and chrome-plated fittings.

CHAPTER NINE

THE MEDICAL-LEGAL AUTOPSY

The application of the autopsy to medical-legal problems, often called the forensic autopsy, should be at least minimally familiar to everyone. So many dramas, detective stories, and other aspects of our culture revolve around unexplained deaths, whether accidental, homicidal, or suicidal, that the person unfamiliar with the autopsy as it is most necessarily applied to these problems must be rare indeed. A popular television series, *Quincy* repeatedly depicts the autopsy room, although understandably, the body on the autopsy table is never shown. Incidentally, one of my principal objections to the show is the introductory portion, showing strong policemen fainting at the sight of the autopsied body; this is totally unrealistic and only serves to reinforce prejudice against the autopsy procedure.

I had originally thought of titling this chapter, "Getting Away With Murder," because by manipulating the various factors which tend to prevent the performance of autopsy, it should be possible for a person with average intelligence to get away with murder. For a death to be investigated properly, there must be someone with a suspicious mind to raise questions. Sometimes a family member questions the cause and nature of a death; but society needs more protection than a dependence on such a hit-or-miss situation, so we structure into our system of social controls individuals whose job it is to be suspicious. Such individuals may be described as detectives, coroners, or medical examiners.

Another important medical-legal aspect of the autopsy is the positive identification of the body. Who was the deceased? Is the deceased the person everyone thinks? Dental charts and other records are useful, but often a complete autopsy is needed to correlate the body with the known facts of the life of the person who the deceased is thought to be. Indeed, a new and growing field is that of forensic anthropology, wherein the practitioner is skilled in interpreting limited findings to infer details that most pathologists can't know from the body at hand. For instance, the forensic anthropologist may be called to determine the sex, stature, and other details from a single thighbone, with the hope that the findings may be fitted with the characteristics of a missing person. Relatively few pathologists, even those with extensive forensic training are equipped to perform this function, but there are experts available in most areas to help the pathologist with a sticky case. Most of the time, however, the pathologist can confirm the identity of the individual, or in the case of a truly unknown body, establish by means of autopsy a volume of details which can be used at some later date to prove the identity by correlation with the characteristics of someone previously known as a "missing person."

There are two ways to consider the medical-legal autopsy: what ought to be done, and what is done. Perhaps I should take the second question first.

There is tremendous variation in the autopsy investigation of death, not only all over the world, but within the United States, and, surprisingly, within many of the states themselves. Some states have excellent, unified, standardized procedures, while others are disorganized, inefficient, variable, and downright dangerous to society. The whole problem in the United States arises from the wisdom of our founding fathers, who specified that all questions not answered by the Constitution are reserved for each state to answer in its own way. The obvious result is much diversity and disorganization and there's not even a federal support program of significance, whereby the central government can bring pressure for uniformity and standardization by withholding funds, a technique which has been successful in bringing the various states in conformity with one another in so many other fields.

FROM THE DESK OF . . .

W.R. BETTY

6 June 16

Hi Frank

Pls. pass this on
to someone who
might enjoy some
lite medical reading

Warren

238
31

Every state of this nation accepts in principle that unexplained deaths must be investigated. So much is inherited from English common law, which is generally the basis of a state's legal system. But then each state apparently feels that it must overlay common law principles with various statutes, and with fifty different legislatures writing the laws, it is not surprising that there is great diversity, and a wide variation in the medical-legal procedures in use here and there. Not that diversity is bad by itself; indeed, many states have programs that are better than could have been written nationally, but there are also more states that have procedures that are terribly inadequate.

Historically, English law created the office of coroner, whose original function was to protect the interest of the Crown in the settlement of the estate of any deceased citizen. From there, it was only a short step to the job of investigating unexplained deaths, since these particularly were often the cases where the interest of the Crown was unclear. Then to the coroner's duties were added the resolution of deaths from criminal, or at least suspect, activity. These the duties of the coroner today.

Many jurisdictions still have coroners, either elected or appointed, who are lawyers, undertakers, druggists, or other persons who, for all their earnest concern for the satisfactory performance of the job, are not trained to handle the problems with which they are faced, problems in which medical knowledge — and specialized medical knowledge — is often necessary. I'm sure that there are many exceptions to this general rule; there must be many who, through careful self-education, have prepared themselves to perform splendidly, but the vast bulk of coroners are just not equipped to handle all phases of medical-legal investigation. Other states have instituted medical examiners who are doctors, but with no special training in forensic medicine, and the result is only slightly better than the coroner system.

On the other hand, there are some states which have superbly organized and integrated systems, with direction by a chief medical examiner who has a law degree as well as an M.D., extensive training in pathology, and special training and certification in forensic pathology from the American Board of Pathology. He has with him a team of pathologists (generally with forensic training), detectives, toxicologists, sociologists, statisticians and other specialists to assist him, and he has the enthusiastic support of the legislature and court system. His office is in charge of every case of death that is appropriate (and we'll get to the definition of the "medical-legal case" in a little while). He makes a determination of the cause and nature of each death, and reports to the state attorney's office on his findings. His office also collects statistics whereby trends of particular types of death can be identified, and important conclusions reached. An example of the importance of statistical studies is seen with the legionnaires' disease discovery a few years ago, as discussed in chapter five. This important problem was not discovered until someone noticed a clustering of cases of death. The disease might well have been identified many years before if there had been careful statistical treatment of deaths on a nationwide basis.

Some states have, over the years, seen the error of their ways and replaced their coroner systems with medical examiner systems. The first state to do this was Massachusetts, which in 1876 found it could no longer live with an inadequate system. The result was splendid for its day: medical examiners were doctors in the community, removed from politics by a five-year governor's appointment, adequately paid for their work, and, by the standards of the day, well-trained to make an accurate determination of the cause of death. The problem in the state a hundred years later, was that no changes had been made since 1876 with the result that many communities became covered only by general practice physicians who had insufficient special training, inadequate pay, and only peripheral interest in the work. Many other jurisdictions were without anyone at all because no one had been appointed to these vacant positions. And there was no central agency to collect statistics. At the time, I was president of the Massachusetts Society of Pathologists. A highly competent general practitioner who was our local medical examiner (and for whom I had done many autopsies) was president of the Massachusetts Association of Medical Examiners. We put our heads together and started the work that has resulted in a new structure, with a chief medical examiner and an office for collection of statistics. Massachusetts now has a modern, efficient medical-examiner system.

One thing that a forensic pathologist is not, whatever his title (medical examiner, coroner, etc.) is a policeman. The picture of the medical examiner who tracks down the murderer may make for good television drama, but it is not good forensic pathology. The conscientious pathologist is, first and always, the servant of truth. I have discussed this elsewhere, but the principle is doubly true in forensic pathology. He must not be an arm of the police or partisan with the district attorney's office. Conversely, he should never be an adversary of these offices. To do his job properly, he must be responsible only to the truth in a particular matter and must let the chips fall where they may. The police and the prosecutors have their functions, and it only destroys the function of the medical examiner if he tries to step into their field.

Now, consider this question. If you wanted to commit murder, would you choose an area with an antiquated coroner system, or one with an organized medical-legal investigative team? The answer is obvious. There are many jurisdictions in this country where you would not have to be half-smart to get away with murder, quite literally. I'm not gong to tell where these are, nor am I going to suggest methods of murder that are most likely to go undiscovered. But the fact remains that, in all too many places, the investigation of possible murder is undertaken only after pressure is brought by relatives or other interested parties, and when such investigation is instituted, it is done so incompetently that murder after murder goes unsolved and unpunished. Once in a while, the authorities will move ahead without being pushed, if there is money involved or if some individual appears to benefit greatly by the death, but these cases are relatively rare. The most frequent type of murder today is that of a senile man or woman kept in the home, unhappy, foul-smelling, and totally out of touch with surroundings and people. Someone in the family decides that enough is enough and adds some rat poison to his food. The doctor is called and signs the death certificate as senile arteriosclerotic heart disease — and murder goes undetected unless someone in the family raises a question.

Even with a well-organized medical-examiner department, things can go wrong, generally because of an overloaded system. I remember a particular case in point from a major city. The police had been called to an apartment where the dead body of a forty-seven-year-old lawyer had been discovered. Death had occurred several days before, and because of the unpleasant odor the police had spent as little time as possible in the room, but reported that there were no marks on the body, no sign of a struggle, and nothing apparently missing from the apartment. The medical examiner, a trained forensic pathologist, was notified, and he sent the local health department physician, a general practitioner with no forensic training, to view the body and certify the death if he saw no problem. The doctor did visit, very briefly because of the odor, and gave a certificate of death due to natural causes, a heart attack. The undertaker was called, and placed the body in a sealed plastic bag. There were no relatives who wished a funeral, so the body was buried promptly without embalming, and without opening the body bag — and the case was closed. It was closed only until a young man was arrested for unauthorized use of credit cards in a distant state, and it was found that the credit cards were those of the deceased. Then things happened. The police investigated, and since the source of the odor had been removed, now spent some time in the apartment. They found the television and stereo missing, and other clear evidences of robbery. The body was then exhumed and autopsied, and the cause of death was immediately apparent. There was a white silk scarf tightly tied around the victim's neck. His heart was fine. The young man was convicted of murder. The medical examiner was roasted by the public press, but the fault really lay in the fact that the medical examiner's department of this large city was so overworked that this case slipped by.

The case we've just discussed brings us, at last, to the subject of this chapter: the medical-legal autopsy and its characteristics. The forensic or medical-legal autopsy has somewhat different objectives than the general type of hospital autopsy. The purpose is not just to study the disease which caused the death but to uncover the manner of death with the object of determining whether or not there is a matter of legal interest involved.

The hospital autopsy is performed with a hospital chart at hand, and the hour-by-hour events leading up to the death are conscientiously recorded. With the forensic autopsy, the investigator is seeking not just why death occurred, but also how. It does not mean that criminal action is necessarily suspected, but only that there is a public interest involved. The case may end up in civil courts, or there is a quasi-judicial board such as workmen's compensation with an interest. For instance, I autopsied a case of a man who injured his hand at work, and was invalided home for a week by the company physician. He was found dead in his own backyard several days later, and the question arose on whether the death was caused by the injury at work, and therefore compensable by the workmen's compensation insurance carried by the employer. Autopsy revealed a longstanding narrowing of a coronary artery branch, and a recent thrombus (clot) completely blocking the artery, causing the heart attack. Here the autopsy served to clarify that the death was not work-connected, and the public was protected from a cost that would have contributed to higher compensation insurance rates.

The converse is just as important. The individual should also be assisted in collection of compensation if it is his right. When accidental death is suspected, an autopsy is quite necessary for the collection of the double-indemnity benefit which is written into so many insurance policies. Cases of apparent suicide should always be autopsied to determine underlying disease as well as to document the case, particularly if there is a clause in the applicable insurance ruling out coverage if suicide occurs within two years of taking out the policy.

Medical-legal autopsy is often necessary for the protection of the innocent. There was a case of a woman who reported taking an overdose of medication. Her psychiatrist told her not to worry because the amount of the drug she had taken was not enough to cause trouble. She then became involved in a fight with her husband, who struck her several times and left the house, returning later to find her dead. He called the police and confessed to murder, but the autopsy showed not only that his blows had inflicted only superficial injury, but also that the poor lady had interpreted the psychiatrist's statement as a hint, and ingested the medication this time in sufficient quantity to kill herself. Without the autopsy, the remorseful husband would still be serving time in the penitentiary.

I believe it is obvious that autopsy is essential in the handling of epidemic diseases, and the medical-legal route is the only way to go to be assured of obtaining the necessary information. And likewise, the study of environmental hazards requires that medical-legal autopsies be performed on all cases of death. Aircraft accident investigation is another area where an autopsy ordered by the authorities is absolutely necessary, and has contributed greatly to the constantly improving record of safety in the air. Fatal automobile accidents must also be investigated for questions of alcohol, drugs, and disease contributing to the accident. These are only a few of many types of death that need to be studied for the protection of the public and for the further development of public polices to prevent tragedy.

Often, the medical-legal autopsy can be used to identify causes of death from which the public can or should be protected. Many of the standards we have for occupational safety have resulted from the autopsies of persons killed at work. The identification of fine particles of silica in the lungs of foundry workers and hard-rock miners has led to stringent requirements for the protection of these workers, and the use of asbestos to coat structural steel has been outlawed on the basis of autopsies which showed that asbestos fragments can cause many tumors of the lungs and related organs.

Protection from other hazards can be developed by the use of the autopsy. I recall one case which I examined where a young man was painting a house, using an aluminum ladder. As he moved from one area to another, the ladder touched an electric wire and he was electrocuted. Autopsy ruled out heart attack or any other cause, and confirmed the effect of electricity. As a result, people are now warned to use wooden or fiberglass ladders, or to use extreme caution; this is not a hazard that can be legislated against, but it does give a chance to issue warning statements.

Most unfortunately, many people never seem to grow up, and industrial plants and other work situations often have individuals who feel they must engage in horseplay and practical jokes. Many deaths have resulted from such activities, and the autopsy is needed to demonstrate the nature of the damage done by such playfulness. An instance comes to mind where a pathologist friend of mine was engaged by the medical examiner to perform an autopsy. This was the case of a young man working as an auto mechanic. While he was bent over the workings of an automobile, one of his coworkers thought it would be funny to "goose" him, but instead of merely ramming his finger between the victim's buttocks, he thought it would much funnier to use the compressed-air hose which was readily available. The victim screamed, collapsed, and promptly died. Autopsy revealed that his entire rectum was ripped to shreds and many major arteries were lacerated. I do not know what happened to the jokester, but I feel he should have been given a long jail term, as a lesson to others who might be tempted to repeat his prank.

Before medical school I was employed briefly as a fisheries biologist in a major fishing port, and part of my job involved working around the moving belts where workers processed the fish, cutting the flesh away from the bones (filleting). These men use very sharp knives, and there was the usual amount of horseplay, in throwing pieces of fish flesh and chunks of ice around, but there was one unwritten rule rigidly observed, that no one raised a knife in anger or in playfulness. To make a gesture that could be interpreted as threatening, with a knife in hand, resulted in the permanent loss of a job, not through any administrative action, but by the other workers themselves. They would not work with anyone foolish enough to underevaluate the important tool of their trade, the knife. Social pressure is effective in these cases, and thankfully, deaths and their consequent autopsies can be prevented.

Perhaps the saddest of deaths which must be carefully investigated is the infant death, whether from disease, trauma, or unknown causes like the Sudden Infant Death Syndrome, or crib death.

Much has been made in the public press about this latter problem, and the impression has been given that the bulk of deaths of children up to six months of age are unexplained. The reverse is true. Careful autopsy results in a clear explanation of most infant deaths. The story is familiar. The child is found dead in his crib without explanation and the medical examiner is told that there is another crib death. But careful inquiry often reveals that the child was fussy, and had a runny nose at bedtime, and autopsy reveals a well-developed pneumonia. Or inquiry shows that the child was found caught down in a fold of the mattress, tightly twisted in a sheet, or pinned by the neck between slats or a broken crib-side, and the autopsy shows the findings of asphyxiation (but "smothered in a pillow" doesn't happen, except in extraordinary circumstances). A certain percentage of apparent crib deaths are actually murders, and autopsy shows the characteristics bruises and burns of child abuse. Nevertheless, a small percentage of autopsies in this group will show no identifiable cause of death, and must be classified as true Sudden Infant Death Syndrome (SIDS). And here the autopsy is particularly important, if only to relieve the guilt feelings of the parents. It is very characteristic of these cases that the parents are consumed by thoughts of what could have been done, and how they are at fault. Sometimes they are at fault, but most SIDS cases cannot have been anticipated, and the family must be reassured that there was nothing they could have done to prevent the death.

The medical-legal autopsy has characteristics which separate it from the hospital autopsy. First, the permission of the next-of-kin is not sought; the autopsy is performed by the order of the coroner, medical examiner or district attorney, depending upon the applicable state law, and the next-of-kin cannot interfere with the procedure short of obtaining a court injunction alleging some misconduct of the official ordering the autopsy. Indeed, it is improper for family permission to be asked unless the interest of the medical examiner has been waived, for fear that family refusal followed by an ordered autopsy might put the medical examiner in a bad light.

Ordinarily, the cases which are M.E. (medical examiner) cases are sudden and unexpected deaths not under medical care (including care of such short duration that the attending doctor has not had time to make a firm diagnosis), deaths from trauma, drugs, radiation exposure or violence, and deaths under any suspicious circumstance. There must also be included any death in police custody, and deaths in the operating room of a hospital. The medical examiner then has to decide whether he can certify the cause of death or if he must order an autopsy. It is remarkable that some medical examiners have such clairvoyance that they rarely order autopsies, while others feel that they need autopsy in somewhere between forty and eighty percent of their cases. The medical examiner can also waive jurisdiction, and the case then reverts to the attending physician for certification of death. This is done fairly frequently in cases that are only technically medical examiner cases, such as one where there was trauma some time before the patient died, but there was a well-established diagnosis not related to the trauma.

In the most efficient systems, the medical examiner is generally a pathologist and conducts his own autopsy, but in other areas, he may be a nonpathologist with the right to hire a pathologist to do the actual examination, in which case he should be with the pathologist throughout the procedure. Before the actual autopsy, there should be a visit to the scene of death, photographs should be taken (sometimes a police photographer will help here), and activities should be performed such as looking for empty medicine bottles, talking with those who may have been present at the time of the fatal episode, and obtaining a health history of the deceased from relatives. Efforts must be made to identify the body by the view of a relative or friend, and confirmation should be sought by studying any identification contained in the pockets of the deceased. The medical examiner should take charge of any money or other objects of value found on the body. The body may then be taken to an autopsy room or a funeral director's preparation room for the actual autopsy.

The autopsy itself is quite similar to the hospital autopsy we've already described, but with a few additional procedures. First, the clothing must be removed, watching for anything unusual, and the body carefully described externally, with photographs as appropriate. Efforts should be made to determine or confirm the time of death; this item is generally known to the minute in a hospital death, but may be of crucial importance in the medical-legal death. Time of death may be determined with fair accuracy by noting the rigor mortis, and the mottling of the body in the lower (dependant) portions, called livor mortis. I object to this latter term because it is inexact and may be misunderstood, since the medical dictionary definition of *livor* includes either deep discoloration or ashen pallor, which are direct opposites. Therefore, I prefer to describe the condition as dependant mottling. Incidentally, if this mottled discoloration is found in other than the more dependant portions, it is evidence that the body has been moved after death. Rigor mortis may vary depending on the temperature of the environment where the body has lain; onset of rigor is generally about six hours after death, beginning with facial muscles and jaw, and passing downward to the leg muscles, and then disappearing in the same order, about eighteen hours after death. The times may be extensively modified, because a body lying in a very warm room may have this sequence quite accelerated, and times may be much slowed if the body is chilled promptly after death.

Determination of the temperature of the body is also a useful procedure in arriving at a likely time of death, and naturally this must be modified by the environment in which the body has lain, but the medical examiner can generally infer a time of death by judging how fast the body lost its heat. I recall a case of double suicide of an elderly brother and sister whose suicide note and other evidence indicated that they died at approximately the same time in a small house without a cellar. The sister's body was found on a bed in an overheated room, and was extensively decomposed, with rigor entirely gone, while the brother was found on the cold tile floor of the adjacent bathroom, with rigor only beginning to be established. Body temperatures were quite different, with the brother's body being very much cooler.

One more item must be taken care of before the autopsy proceeds: if the cause of death appears to be gunshot, the body should be X-rayed before autopsy to determine the location of a bullet if any. The same applies to extensive trauma by metal fragments as in the case of explosion, but in cases without probable bullets or metal fragments, X-ray can be skipped.

The autopsy then proceeds, with careful notes kept throughout (often using a tape recorder), and photographs taken as appropriate. The medical-legal autopsy nearly always includes the head examination, because, if the case lands in court, any lawyer can imply that the examination is worthless because it did not exclude disease of the brain, regardless of what may have been found elsewhere in the body. Generally too, samples of blood are taken for toxicology analysis; these may be sent to the toxicology laboratory right away, or kept (carefully identified) against some unexpected question being raised, no matter what the autopsy apparently showed. Continuity of custody is a watchword on these toxicology specimens. The specimens must be identified and kept under lock in a refrigerator, or, if transferred to another person, receipts must be obtained, all with the purpose of keeping anyone from saying that the specimens were mixed up or deliberately changed.

Toxicology uses blood samples to the best advantage, but many cases need additional specimens either for confirmation of the results of the blood specimens, or in some instances, to determine substances which cannot be precisely analyzed in blood. Samples of bile, for instance, are more useful in determining the presence of some narcotics, and stomach contents may be useful in many cases of poisons taken orally, which have not been fully absorbed into the blood at the time of death. Stomach contents will sometimes show pill remnants, and occasionally complete identifiable pills, making the job of the toxicologist much easier. Often portions of liver, kidney or brain, carefully wrapped in foil and frozen, have been used to identify poisons that could not be determined otherwise. Urine also can be very useful in toxicology, and in some cases, particularly if blood is not available or the toxic substance has disappeared from the blood, it is possible to draw out fluid from the center of the eye for important studies. Cases of drowning should have two blood samples drawn, from the left heart and the right heart, if it is important to determine whether the deceased drowned in fresh or salt water, since fresh water in the lung will draw salt out of the blood (hence a lower level of salt in the left-heart blood) but salt water will add salt, making the level higher in the left specimen. If the salt level is the same, it probably means only that insufficient water was drawn into the lungs before death, not an unusual circumstance.

The odors of the opened body can give the prosector valuable clues, and point to specific diagnoses. For instance, the odor of acetone suggests that the patient died in a diabetic coma. The odor of ingested alcohol is quite distinctive, and quite different from the odor of alcohol in the bottle. Information such as this is very valuable to the toxicologist, who hates to be faced with a request for "general unknowns," because it means many hours of work; a clue given by odor on the most likely rewarding areas of investigation from the prosector could save a great deal of time.

A few rules must be observed in the medical-legal autopsy which are different from the hospital autopsy. It is essential that all unauthorized persons be excluded. The medical-legal autopsy is not the place where medical students and nurses should be permitted to observe, no matter how valuable it would be for the purposes of education. All persons legitimately present should have their names recorded in the record, and all such persons should be admonished that the procedure is of legal significance and is of a confidential nature. Careless public discussion of findings has destroyed the usefulness of many otherwise carefully completed cases.

Bullet wounds are a special problem in some forensic cases, and careful investigation can sometimes, but not always, give important information. If the position of the body at the time of wounding is known, then the direction of the bullet's course can be determined with considerable accuracy by determining the course within the body — but with the possibility of false findings in some cases. Only the experience of the investigator can help in some cases, such as when a bullet hits the inside of a rib and follows it around the body, completely changing the apparent direction. Entrance and exit wounds are sometimes a puzzle. The entrance should be a small round hole with a ring of bruising around it, and the exit wound an irregular hole with radiating laceration of the surrounding skin. But if the muzzle of the gun is held against the skin, then the gases which propel the bullet can follow the bullet into the body and blow back, producing radiating lacerations which look exactly like the exit wound. Powder granules on the skin or the clothing may identify an entrance wound, but again, if the gun is in contact with the skin, the powder granules will all be inside the body. The whole subject of bullet wounds is very complex, and whole books have been written about them. Only the experience of the investigator determines the amount and value of the information derived.

Another problem occurs in military or disaster situations in the identification of individuals found in mass graves. The cause of death may be painfully obvious, but the identity of the victims needs to be established, not only to satisfy the anxieties of the next-of-kin, but also to complete military records and provide documentation for insurance and other purposes. The problem of "missing in action" occurs in many military situations, and remains to plague the settlement of differences when combat is over and attempts are made to establish a workable peace. In these cases, the pathologist often has to call upon the service of a forensic anthropologist to assist him in making positive or tentative identifications.

An example is the situation where a large aircraft crashes and burns behind enemy lines in wartime. The partially incinerated remains of the crew members and passengers are hastily buried in a common grave without formality by the local inhabitants, who keep no record of what was done or when. The mass grave is discovered, months or even years later, and the identification team comes to the scene. At this point, all they have to work with is a pile of unrelated bones. The first problem is to identify just how many bodies do these bones represent, and it has been found that the most reliable way is to count the number of femoral-head structures and divide by two. The femoral head is the upper end of the thighbone, a nearly perfect sphere of bone that forms part of the hip joint; this structure is most readily recognizable and cannot be mistaken, it is less fragile than other bones, and it is often protected from destruction by the cup-like acetabulum of the hip joint.

Often, it is impossible to allocate all the bones to specific pairs of femoral-heads, but many fragments can be associated, jigsaw-puzzle fashion, with the individual pairs to give a good idea of the number of persons buried and a reasonable determination of each skeleton. Indeed, the size of the femoral head itself will give a good clue as to the stature and weight of the individual. A large bone comes from a large person, and the internal structure of the bone can give a good idea about the amount of weight the bone has been supporting. All in all, the team can do a remarkable job of separating the bones into piles representing each individual.

Diligent search for artifacts at the burial site can often turn up some item which will help tremendously in more specific identification. If one dog tag is found, then one body can be matched with it; then if this individual can be identified as a member of a crew of a specific aircraft, the other identities can be established with reasonable certainty by matching the stature and weight determinations with the records of other crew members of that specific aircraft. And so the problem can be solved.

Every reader is probably familiar with the use of dental records to assist in identification. By correlating the teeth of an unidentified body with existing dental records, a practically sure identification can be established. The problems with this are, first: the investigator must have at least a tentative identification in order to know where to start looking. It is manifestly impossible to match an unknown with the literally millions of dental records existing in the world. Second, it is often found that dental records are incomplete or inaccurate, so a perfect match cannot be established. All too often, the dentist performing work on the teeth of an individual may be careless in the completion of his records, or even more often, the patient has visited several dentists, so there is no record which matches exactly the condition found in the dead body. But when a good match is obtained, a precise identification can be made, because there are so many variations in tooth structure and the techniques of repair that the possibility of duplication is practically nonexistent.

Other important features of identification are operative, too. Traumatic scars can be matched with an individual's history or physical examination, and tattoos are particularly useful; indeed, some tattoos will actually have the name of the decedent. Of course, this implies that there is fairly intact skin with which to work, but remarkable things can be done to partially decomposed bodies to bring out scars and tattoos. Even with extensive burning of the body, it is possible to bring out some tattoos by examination under ultraviolet light. Occupational stigmata can also give important clues. Characteristic callouses of the hands may serve to identify the body as that of a tailor, a professional cellist, or some other occupation. A particular paint, dye, or grease under the fingernails may help with identification by suggesting one occupation or another.

Just as with the living person, the fingerprint is often the most useful and rewarding factor in the identification of an unknown body. There are really very few individuals in our culture who have not had fingerprints taken at one time or another, and many of these are in the extensive files maintained by government agencies with computerized classification which can narrow the search from a needle-in-the-haystack situation to a level of practicality. The taking of fingerprints from a dead body is easily done in most cases, and even when there has been extensive burning or other destruction of the fingers, techniques are available which make it possible to determine at least a partial fingerprint in a large number of cases. If the body is shriveled so fingerprints are obscured, the injection of fluid can generally overcome the problem. Often when a body is found floating in water, and fingerprints do not help on the first attempt, the skin may be slipped off the tip of each finger and preserved, for further attempts at identification.

Blood groups can often be determined from very small samples of material — not necessarily blood — with the identification of the A-B-O type, the M-N series, the Rh factors, and many other special groups that exist. The identification of specific antibodies in blood may be matched with items in some individual's history, evidence of previous exposure to measles virus, fungus disease, or other illness to corroborate a tentative identification. All in all, with knowledge of size and weight, sex, race, dental characteristics, blood groups, and many other factors, it is possible to do a good job of identification, and if fingerprints can be matched, then absolute identification can be obtained.

The medical-legal autopsy occupies a very valuable place in the social controls which must exist in order to have a viable civilization, and the efficiency with which such autopsies are obtained and done makes a great difference in how we live. Many examples come to mind on autopsies poorly done, and of cases which should have been autopsied and weren't. On the very day I wrote this chapter, I read in the paper about the suspension of a medical examiner following the exhumation and autopsy of five cases because he certified their deaths as due to natural causes, but the autopsy found bullet wounds and other important causes of death. I will discuss some similar cases involving the autopsy or lack of autopsy of famous persons in chapter fourteen.

CHAPTER TEN

THE AUTOPSY AND RELIGION

Religion has, from prehistoric times, been intimately concerned with death and the disposal of the bodies of its deceased communicants. It is not surprising that there is considerable interaction between religion and the question of autopsy. Autopsy is affected by religious beliefs, and religion is modified to an appreciable degree by the desirability of autopsy. Religious ideas are, in common with all human activity and thought, in a constant state of change as new insights are given to mankind, and therefore, over the many years of recorded history, the impact of religion on autopsy and of autopsy on religion, are constantly altering the social situation. Constant unswerving loyalty to the "faith of our fathers" is in many ways admirable, but unreasonable rigidity even in the most orthodox of religions is not, and the case may be made that such rigidity is self-destructive; the religion that cannot adapt to changing social conditions is doomed to disappear. Religious attitudes which speak to the problems surrounding the autopsy of the dead body have changed considerably over the years.

Religion has quite rightly surrounded death with appropriate procedures aimed at the proper, respectful disposal of the body, and at satisfying the need of the survivors for the exercise of grief — a very necessary procedure for mental health. Sometimes the rules devised to carry out these purposes can interfere with the legitimate purposes of medical investigation, mostly through a misapplication of the religious principles involved or through rules that, when originally instituted, could not envisage the autopsy procedure because it had never been developed.

Sometimes, very regrettably, religion is used as the excuse for real anti-intellectualism. There is a tendency to reject that which we cannot understand, and those who do not understand the need for autopsy sometimes appeal to religion as the excuse for its rejection. I believe that I can demonstrate in this chapter that, among the world's religions, there is no valid objection to the autopsy procedure, and that those who appeal to religion as an excuse for interfering with the investigation of the causes of death through the autopsy are misinterpreting the religion they profess.

The predominant religious concept in America and Europe is obviously the Christian tradition, but with so many variations that some sects are scarcely recognizable as belonging to the same general group. But all Christians look to the teachings of Jesus of Nazareth, as variously recorded and interpreted for their central body of thought. While there is nothing in the Christian scriptures which speaks directly to the question of autopsy, one thing that all Christian thinkers apparently agree on is that the body is but dust and should return to dust; the spirit is the essential divine part of the individual, and when the spirit has left the body, the body is no longer of any religious significance.

Roman Catholicism sees the body of a deceased person as deserving of respect, and it generally rules against cremation, although this does not appear to be basic, and seems likely to be changed before too long. Catholicism has always been able to change to fit changing conditions, and it seems likely that it will respond to the increasing unavailability of land for burial purposes. The Roman Church has supported the use of autopsy for a thousand years, at first reluctantly and with much opposition from church leaders, but when Pope Alexander died suddenly in 1410 autopsy was performed, and Pope Sixtus IV formally sanctioned dissection of human bodies at Bologna and Padua about 1480.

As noted in chapter two, many of the early pathologists were monks, priests, or persons otherwise officially connected with the Roman Church, and through the subsequent years there has been ecclesiastical support for autopsies. After all, the Church has been a leader in the care of the sick, and combined with rational approach to human problems which has characterized Catholic thinking over the years, it is not surprising that there is such support.

One difficulty is the religious question of the physical resurrection of the body on the Day of Judgment, and it has been a concern among some Catholic authorities that all parts of the body be buried together in consecrated ground. This has been carried to the point of burial of an amputated leg in the plot where the rest of the body will lie, some time in the future. The practice of incineration of the viscera after completion of the autopsy has been criticized by some officials of the Church, but all of my Roman Catholic pathologist friends seem to have no hesitation about sending the viscera to the incinerator, so I conclude that this is not a compelling problem.

The open casket funeral seems to be the predominant practice among American Catholics, and this is often preceded by a wake, where the body is displayed to the mourners. But as I will show in chapter eleven, there is nothing to preclude autopsy in such cases, since the autopsy properly done leaves no external marks which can be seen with the clothed body in a casket.

Protestant Christianity, with its wide range of divergent sects, is widely divided in opinions and practices relating to the performance of autopsy. The fundamentalist sects, with a predominance of primitive emotionalism, are frequently uneasy about autopsy, but generally do not interfere when the importance of the autopsy is explained. The objection within this group is not on any appeal to scripture, but rather on the level of a non-intellectual or even anti-intellectual feeling. It is largely this same group that turns to faith healers and naturopaths, so it is not surprising that they decline to cooperate with mainstream doctors and pathologists when postmortem examination is requested.

The conformist group of Protestant religionists tends to come to the same conclusion as the Catholics, but are more inclined to grant autopsy permission because they are generally a somewhat more highly educated group, and the granting of autopsy permission seems to be more associated with the level of education than with any religious feelings. The more liberal Christians and intellectual sects among the Protestants seem eager for autopsies to be done, and it is not unusual for members of these groups to request or even demand autopsies when the procedure is not offered to them.

Judaism is quite a different problem. While there is no prohibition of dissection of the dead body among Christians, there is a definite body of Jewish law which is all too often interpreted as ruling out autopsy permission. The Hebrew leaders who initiated these rules deserve high marks for sensitive humanitarianism, because they were ruling against the dishonoring of the dead body. The concept apparently arose at a time when members of other ethnic groups would tie the body of a defeated enemy to the tail of a chariot and drag it in the dust, or dismember or disembowel the body of the defeated to celebrate a victory. Such activity is repulsive, and we can be glad for the sensitive reaction of the Jewish people.

"Judaism always considered the body sacred," states Rabbi Max Drob. "The human body, the Bible tells us, was fashioned by God Himself, who created Man in his own image and appointed the body as the abode of the soul." This attitude looks to Deuteronomy 21:22–23 which states, "And if a man have committed a sin worthy of death, and he is to be put to death, and thou hang him on a tree; his body shall not remain all night upon the tree, but thou shalt in any wise bury him that day." The implication, according to Jewish interpretation, is that, if a criminal is to be given such respect, how much more should we respect the body of an average man. The scholarly Jewish comments on this passage state that a disgrace (*nivul*) of the body is forbidden to Jews.

On the other hand, about 100 A.D., Rabbi Ismael is said to have permitted the body of an executed prostitute to be boiled to remove the flesh, so that an accurate count of the bones of the body could be made. Jewish scholarship has frequently been at odds with Jewish religiosity, and there are many similar instances where scholarship has been held to be more important than the strict application of religious rules.

The range of modern interpretation of this idea is quite wide with some orthodox rabbis ruling that any dissection of the body is a *nivul.* Indeed, a number of passages of the Talmud speak specifically of an autopsy as a disgrace to the body and absolutely forbidden. But rabbinical thought in many other instances leads to the conclusion that an exception should be made in cases where autopsy might result in the saving of human life — and here again we find a difference of interpretation. Some rabbis rule that saving the of life of a specific individual in the community suffering from the same disease that caused the death in question is the only case that justifies an autopsy. Others feel that, with today's scientific publication and rapid communication, the whole world is a community and that, consequently, autopsy can be permitted quite generally because autopsy findings will indeed aid in saving some human life somewhere; there is no need to have a specific person in mind.

The most successful rejoinder to the argument that autopsy is a disgrace and therefore forbidden by Jewish law is that there is no disgrace, no disrespect for the body of the deceased. Indeed, the autopsy is intended as a positive act of respect for the body of the deceased, and I would even go so far as to say that it dishonors the body to bury it without autopsy. It is unquestionable that the conscientious pathologist, no matter if the particular autopsy is the thousandth in his career, approaches the autopsy with respect for the body and for the knowledge which is to be gained. As I stated in an earlier chapter, I have never done an autopsy where I didn't encounter some interesting variation, some new item, or some other fact that made that particular autopsy different from all others and rewarding in new knowledge. The result is that I have always had respect for the body and what it can teach me, and I believe most pathologists, Jew or gentile, perform autopsies with the same respect.

Perhaps another answer which might be even more telling, when Jewish prohibition of autopsies is cited, is the fact that in the state of Israel, where the profound influence of the religious authorities is undeniable, every hospital death is routinely autopsied. No permission of the next-of-kin is required, and indeed it is very difficult to prevent the hospital pathologists from performing an autopsy. Hospital admission implies consent for autopsy, and autopsy is done regardless of any opposition from the interpreters of Jewish law.

Islam shares with Christianity the heritage from the ancient Hebrew culture, and in many ways it is quite similar in its basic opinion regarding autopsy. There is no specific prohibition of autopsy in the Koran, and one of the basics of Islam is that the Koran and the teachings of Mohammed are the final, definitive revelation, with only very limited room for interpretation. Since there is no comment in these sources, then there can be no religious opposition to the procedure. There is, however, especially among the more primitive adherents of the faith, a revulsion against the opening of the dead body, as there is in most primitive groups. The result, in some Muslim countries, is that there is intense objection to the performance of autopsies on the part of tribal organizations, which are a very potent social force in these countries. This objection is often couched in religious terms, and is supported by the religious authorities who are at some pains not to offend the tribal organizations.

I have talked recently with an American pathologist who had just returned from a period of teaching and practice in Saudi Arabia. He told me of the case of a prominent Arab citizen who expired, and of the Western-educated nephew of the deceased who was a physician and who urgently desired an autopsy, since the cause of death was not clear. It so happened that the pathologist was scheduled for home leave to the United States, so he proceeded to do the autopsy before his departure, with the knowledge of the nephew but without informing anyone else. Then he left for America the next morning. When he returned to his duties two months later, things had calmed down, but the nephew told him that if he hadn't gone away, he would very likely have been kidnapped by the members of the tribe of the deceased and stoned to death. And the civil authorities would not have interfered at all. The civil authorities, on the other hand, had no basis for action against him, and he completed a successful tour of duty.

Other countries with large Islamic populations vary considerably from Saudi Arabs, but in none of them is found any real religious objection to autopsy. The only problem seems to be the support which conservative religious authorities often give to groups with primitive, anti-intellectual feelings, and this appears to be a problem with all religions of the world.

Dr. Samuel McClatchie of New Zealand tells of his service in Malawi, a predominantly Moslem country. He had been asked to do a medical-legal autopsy by the local police, but was confronted by an angry group of upcountry natives protesting the procedure. "If you do the autopsy, they will kill you, " reported his diener. So Dr. McClatchie called the police, who took the angry group away. They returned an hour later, agreeing to the autopsy. Later, he asked the diener how they were persuaded to change their minds. "The police beat them," was the answer. This seems hardly an acceptable way to get an autopsy permission, but apparently it was effective in this case.

Buddhism, the fourth-most prominent religion of the world from the point of view of the total number of adherents (Christianity, Islam, and Hinduism have larger numbers) likewise has no objection to the postmortem examination of the body. Indeed, it is quite aloof from such concerns since the basic idea of Buddhism is that life is misery and decay, and that there is no ultimate reality in it or behind it. Since "self" is unreal and the endless cycle of birth and rebirth continues only because of desire, it is not surprising that there is nothing said about autopsy, which is directed toward relief of misery, toward prolongation of life, and in a sense, toward the gratification of desire. While Buddhism has nothing to say about autopsy, it is quite understandable that its philosophy could lead to a lack of sympathy for, and even opposition to autopsy.

In actual practice, autopsy is performed rarely in those countries lying along the southern border of Asia from India to Japan, with large Buddhist populations; this is not from any specific impact of religion, but more from a combination of otherworldliness of the educated religious leaders, and from an appalling lack of education and intellectual concern in the great body of people adherent to this religion.

Hinduism, like Buddhism, suffers from a widespread lack of education among most of its communicants, and a fatalism which leads to a profound lack of interest in life-preserving and disease-preventing measures of which autopsy of the dead body plays such a significant part. Many of the hospitals and other health facilities of India where this form of religion is most prevalent are operated under the auspices of a Christian minority who seek to improve the quality of life; but today there is evidence of a growing interest in change, and an increase in the number of physicians and other health-care personnel trained in the Hindu community.

It is probably fair to say that there is no specific objection to autopsy within the Hindu tradition, and there is growing support for the procedure coming from young Hindu physicians who are grappling with the severe health problems of their area. Indeed, the care of sickness is one of the pure acts to which the devout Hindu is called, and I believe there will be an increasing involvement with health care in the Hindu community, accompanied by increasing support of the autopsy procedure.

About the remaining predominant religions of the world, there is little to say. Shinto, Confucian, and Taoist groups are little different from the Buddhist community with which they coexist, with respect to autopsy and general concepts of health care. While there is no specific opposition to autopsy in these religions, there is no enthusiastic support for concepts of health care and for educated investigation into the causes of disease.

What can be said of the impact of atheism on the concern of autopsy? Atheism, which is found in all areas of the world but with official sanction in only a few, appears not to interfere with autopsy in most of its expressions, and since it is generally intellectual in form, it tends to give considerable support to the concept. There is no afterlife or physical resurrection to consider in this philosophy, so this primitive objection to the dissection of the body is removed. Since many atheists of the past reached their beliefs through education and philosophical thought, it is not surprising that there is real support for autopsy among atheists. I hope that this fact will not be seized upon by religionists to excuse their objections to autopsy, saying that, since atheists are for the idea, it must be wrong. If Adolph Hitler was in favor of taking baths, would it mean that we must not take baths? Such stupidity is anti-intellectualism in its worst form, and should not be tolerated.

All in all, it can be stated that there is no legitimate religious objection to autopsy in any of the religion which are prevalent in he world. No religion can claim a real opposition to the investigation of the causes of death, and the dissection of the bodies of the dead as part of that investigation. Only Judaism comes close to such an objection, and even this needs not be a compelling objection. The resistance to autopsy, sometimes presented in religious terms, appears to come almost entirely from a primitive fear of the dead body and what it represents, in reminding us of our own mortality.

CHAPTER ELEVEN

THE AUTOPSY AND THE FUNERAL DIRECTOR

In many communities, the relationship between pathologists and funeral directors is characterized by great tension and animosity, while in other communities, there is earnest professional cooperation. Why is there a difference? It seems to depend on how much effort each of these professional groups is willing to make in understanding the problems and attitudes of the other. There is a very wide difference between the objectives of the pathologist and the funeral director. The pathologist, as mentioned earlier, is concerned with the study of disease and its effects on the anatomy of the body.

The funeral director, on the other hand, is deeply involved in a relationship with the next-of-kin during the very difficult emotional time that follows the death of a loved one. In the United States, where the open casket is often on display during the visiting hours and sometimes also at the funeral, the appearance of the body is of prime importance, and it is understandable that the funeral director takes a dim view of the interference with the integrity of the body implicit in the work of the pathologist. Incidentally, the nursing profession is also quite properly concerned with the appearance of the body of the patient in life, hence the uneasiness that is often expressed by nurses when the question of autopsy comes up. The cleanliness of the body is of great importance to nurses and to funeral directors as well; it must be admitted that some pathologists are not as careful as they should be in seeing that the body appears clean and neat when it is turned over to the undertaker after an autopsy.

I want to state at the outset that the funeral director is, or at least should be, a professional in the best sense of the word. Historically the professions have been seen to be those occupations primarily concerned with service to humanity, with remuneration for services only a secondary consideration; the ministry, medicine, and the law were the three occupations generally listed as professions, but I feel that the calling of the funeral director is among the occupations which should be included as well. There are, of course, examples of individuals who fail to live up to the high standards of a profession in every group, and certainly there are, among funeral directors, many individuals whose performance fails to qualify. The real professional funeral director is the one who is available to shoulder the burden of the many things which must be done, and done promptly, when death has occurred and the family of the deceased is in understandable emotional tension and confusion. He is the man who knows what must be done, and is prepared to do it; a good funeral director is a blessing to be accepted with gratitude.

It has become a common attitude in some segments of our culture to regard the funeral director as a parasite on society, praying on the bereaved family at a time when its members are most vulnerable and distressed. Jessica Mitford's book, *The American Way of Death*, is one of the outstanding examples of this attitude. Sad to relate, this criticism is unquestionably accurate concerning some undertakers. The urge to sell the most costly coffin, to imply that a concrete vault liner is required by law, and to add on charges for unnecessary services turns the funeral home into a for-profit business. A professional would offer these services, state those that are not legally necessary, and leave the choice to the family. He would state that even embalming is not required by law, and that it can be dispensed with if the body is refrigerated or is disposed of promptly. All too often, however, the undertaker will suggest, if not state directly, that it is somehow disrespectful to the deceased not to spend heavily for the unessential portions of the funeral activity in spite of limited funds, and under this unnecessary pressure some families have been truly impoverished by funeral costs. The professional funeral director should seek out the family's desires, and discourage unnecessary expenditures when family funds are limited.

In my work as a medical examiner's pathologist, I was called on frequently to take my kit of autopsy instruments to the preparation room of a funeral home to perform an autopsy on the body of an individual who had died under suspicious, or at least confusing, circumstances. In chapter nine, I dealt with the medical-legal autopsy, but here, I wish only to point out that working in embalmers' preparation rooms over the years gave me extensive contact with a number of widely different funeral homes. And when I was chief of laboratory service in a Veterans Administration hospital, one of my duties was to inspect the premises, equipment, and personnel of funeral homes bidding on contracts to handle funerals for deceased veterans, which are offered to families at government expense. As a result, I got to know the characteristics of a good funeral home, and I saw a lot of bad ones.

Some funeral establishments have beautifully-appointed parlors and other rooms which are seen by the public, but miserable, dirty closets that serve as preparation rooms where the embalming, and sometimes a medical-legal autopsy, must be done. Other funeral homes have scrupulously clean, well-lighted embalming rooms which could serve as operating rooms in an emergency, not that any surgeon would like to operate in such a room; no matter how clean, the embalming area must always be regarded as contaminated, and suitable precautions observed. The conscientious funeral director and his embalmer are acutely conscious of the hazards of bacterial and viral diseases, and treat their preparation room accordingly. If death has occurred in a hospital, bodies of those who have died of infectious disease are generally labeled by a yellow tag or other device and extra-special precautions are exercised in those cases, but every death should be handled as if dangerous infection were present because sometimes it is, even when it was not suspected before death. Many a case of death by heart attack may also have some disease like tuberculosis, for instance, and the people handling the body must protect themselves against infection by treating every case as if it were highly contagious. The handling of bodies of those who have died following treatment with radioactive medications also requires special precautions in the embalming process similar to those I outlined in chapter seven.

I worked in one undertaking establishment which specialized in embalming bodies for other funeral directors (a trade embalmer). In their preparation room I saw bodies stacked up on the floor, one upon another, like so much cordwood, waiting for one of the several embalming tables to be free. Other funeral homes I saw were able to survive on one or two funerals a month; the funeral director would make a living by operating in a big old house no one wanted to live in because of the inordinate expense. He would equip the first floor as funeral parlors, using his own labor to paint, paper, carpet, and so on; the preparation room would usually be in the basement, and he and his family would live upstairs. His wife answered the telephone and did the bookkeeping. When the funeral director did a funeral, he would hire for the job: the hearse, the flower car, the family car, and the heavy equipment needed, as well as the embalmer, the pallbearers and other personnel; and he did make a living.

Jessica Mitford, in her perceptive book, states, "The funeral men hate autopsies." And indeed they often do, but she also admits that the well-trained, conscientious funeral director will often assist in obtaining autopsy permission. "It is generally the badly trained or avaricious undertaker who is resistant to the autopsy procedure," she states, and this is entirely in conformity with my experience.

What must the pathologist know and do, in order to preserve cordial relations with the funeral director? First, he must know that there should be no great delay in releasing the body to the undertaker, so that all the necessary procedures such as embalming, dressing, and casketing may be carried out in an unhurried and thorough manner. All too often, particularly in the large university hospitals, the body is stored in the morgue refrigerator for twenty-four hours or more while permission is being sought — or sometimes not being sought because the responsible physician is too busy attending to the living to spend time concerned with the dead. Or sometimes the doctor who must get the autopsy permission is emotionally blocked; he doesn't want to face the fact of the failure of his therapy, so he drags his feet and puts the interview with the next-of-kin at the end of his other duties. After all, getting an autopsy permission is often a real selling job, and doctors are often not very good salesmen.

In other cases, delay may be directly caused by the pathologist himself. He may be too busy with his other duties, or he may not understand the needs of the funeral director for prompt release of the body.

Sometimes the delay is caused by bureaucratic red tape in the administration of the hospital, or by lack of communication between various departments of the hospital. Many times I have sent word that my autopsy was complete, but the message was lost and did not reach the person who could release the body. The funeral director, meanwhile, is forced to wait, while the anxious family pressures him to commit himself about the time for visiting hours, and for the funeral itself. The delay, no fault of his, is deeply embarrassing to him, and interferes with his duty to support the family psychologically. It prevents the smooth arrangements that the family of the deceased has every right to expect.

Sometimes delay in the release of a body is caused, not by the attending doctor, the pathologist, or the hospital administration, but by the medical examiner. In cases of unexplained or suspicious deaths like those considered in chapter nine, the medical examiner must make out the death certificate; and he will not do this, and often not even authorize the moving of the body, until the public interest which he is charged with protecting is satisfied. As a result, a body may be held for several days, generally under refrigeration, and the funeral director gets frustrated and angry. But there is no way to prevent this short of obtaining a court order, which no judge should issue unless he is satisfied that the medical examiner has caused the delay through laziness, malice or incompetence.

The medical examiner may also cause delay in cases where the body is to be cremated. Most states require that a body for cremation be held, refrigerated if possible, or sometimes embalmed with permission of the medical examiner, for forty-eight hours, should there appear any problem which might suggest the need of autopsy for medical-legal reasons. The medical examiner must then certify that he has no further interest in the case before cremation can take place. Obviously, a buried body can be exhumed if medical-legal questions arise after the death and burial, but a jar of ashes can rarely answer any questions. This necessary policy may delay the work of the funeral director, and contribute to unfriendly feelings among the professional people and the families involved.

The pathologist himself may be directly responsible for another problem which can cause trouble for the funeral director. This is the performance of the autopsy in a way which so affects the body that the open-casket display of the body, desired by many families in our culture, is interfered with. The autopsy might be done so that embalming becomes very difficult, or even impossible, or worse, the pathologist may make incisions in the face or hands which are impossible to conceal. The ordinary technique described in chapter three places the skin incisions where they can be concealed with clothing after the body is dressed and placed in the casket. If the brain has been included in the autopsy, the incision can be placed where the hair may be combed over it, and even a bald head may be autopsied satisfactorily if the incision is placed far at the back of the head so that it may be concealed by a fluffed pillow. Occasionally, however, a poorly instructed prosector may make an incision across the forehead, or in his zeal to understand a particular disease, so damage the nose, eyelids, mouth, or hands that the embalmer cannot reestablish a normal appearance. I would hope that such disfigurement of a body would not be the result of a malicious wish to embarrass the funeral director, but I have heard funeral directors describe damage which is hard to explain except on the basis of malice.

Another complaint that funeral directors direct at some pathologists is the matter of the availability and continuity of the blood vessels which the embalmer must have to do his work properly. The best way to distribute embalming fluid throughout the body is by the use of the body's existing blood vessels. Vascular embalming is almost universally used on the unautopsied body, by running a trocar (essentially a very large gauge hollow needle as much as a quarter-inch in diameter) through the abdominal wall just below the rib cage into the ventricles of the heart and apply suction, to remove the fluid blood. Much of the blood remains fluid after death because the ability of blood to clot, while extensive, is used up before a large amount of the blood is solidified. The embalmer then makes a small incision, often in the armpit or in the anterior shoulder area, to find a blood vessel and injects his embalming fluid under pressure through a smaller needle. The resulting pressure and suction causes the embalming fluid to run through the blood vessels throughout the body and replace the blood, and when the suction on the trocar shows embalming fluid rather than blood, the perfusion is complete. It's not all that easy. The adjustment of the features of the face and many other problems must be solved at the same time, but I'm not writing a treatise on embalming, but rather considering the problems of autopsy in relation to embalming.

When performing an autopsy, the pathologist-prosector must naturally interfere with the blood vessels, so the embalming technique described for the unautopsied body cannot be used. But the autopsy can be done with preservation of the essential blood vessels the embalmer needs. His purposes can be well served if there are the major arteries to the head, neck, arms, and legs available and uninterrupted. To review anatomy for a moment, the blood leaves the heart through the main artery (the aorta) and very soon branches off to other arteries near the center of the first U-turn (three or four inches along its course) known as the arch of the aorta. These branches are called the innominate (no name!), the left common carotid, and the left subclavian. The innominate divides very soon into the right common carotid and the right subclavian, which is perhaps the reason no one wanted to give it a name. The carotids on each side supply blood to the entire head and neck, and the subclavians supply the two arms, so it is easy to see that, if these vessels are intact and available, the embalmer can do the most important parts of his job using these vessels. Indeed, I know one embalmer who, if the arch of the aorta is left in place, places a clamp on either side of the three main branches, and embalms the entire upper part of the body with only one injection site. The embalming fluid is forced in under pressure and flows through the arterial system, eventually running clear out of the cut ends of the veins into the body cavity.

What can the pathologist do to make the embalmer hate him? He can pull down on the carotid arteries (they are quite elastic), and reaching up into the neck with scissors, snip them off as high as he can reach. The cut ends of the arteries will then snap back, away into the uppermost portion of the neck, and the embalmer will be left with no available vessels with which to process the face and neck structures. All he can do is to try to infiltrate the tissues by needle and syringe with embalming fluid, and hope. The job done this way is long and difficult, and the result is generally less than satisfactory.

Similarly, the embalmer needs the arteries leading into the legs — the common iliac vessels which are formed by the final division of the aorta into two vessels — in order to embalm the legs. If the prosector cuts these short, or cuts across them further down in the leg while investigating disease in the leg itself, then he causes the embalmer problems, but not as severe problems as the destruction of the vessels to the head because needle and syringe embalming can be done more quickly and with less worry about the appearance, since the area will be covered in the casket. Indeed, even when the pathologist leaves perfectly adequate vessels, the needle and syringe technique must be used on the flanks, the buttocks, and other areas not served by the vessels already discussed.

Some hospital pathology departments go to considerable lengths to make funeral directors happy. It is quite common to tie off the vessels the embalmer needs, and leave long strings to aid him in finding the vessels. Some hospitals even go so far as to insert glass tubes in the cut ends of the arteries, and connect them with rubber tubing, so that one rubber tube extends outside and the embalmer has only to connect to his machine and embalm the entire body all at once. The ultimate in trying to keep the funeral director happy occurs at one hospital I know of where there is an embalmer on the hospital payroll who embalms the body free of charge before it is released to the undertaker. Regrettably, it has happened in some cases from this hospital that the next-of-kin have been charged for embalming anyway, and the undertaker has pocketed the money.

What about the viscera (the abdominal and thoracic organs) and the brain which have been removed? Some hospitals take them to the incinerator after all the tissue samples have been taken for study, while others place them back in the body. In the former case, there is no problem for the embalmer, and in the latter, the embalmer merely places the organs in a plastic bag with very strong embalming fluid and sews them up in the body for burial. The return of the viscera to the body, except for small fragments used to make the glass slides for study under the microscope, makes the autopsy acceptable to many orthodox Jews and to some other religious groups, when the disposal by incineration would violate their requirement that all parts of the body be buried together in one spot. Some groups go so far as to save hair clippings and fingernail parings to be buried with the body, so it is understandable that incineration of the viscera would be objectionable to them.

Another problem for the embalmer occurs when the family, responding reluctantly to the entreaties for autopsy permission, grants a limited autopsy. Suppose the apparent cause of death is a perforated stomach ulcer, and the family finally consents to an autopsy, limited to the abdominal cavity. This means that the embalmer is faced with a body where the abdominal viscera are out of the way, but he can't get to the head and arm vessels, nor can he efficiently use the technique for an unautopsied body since too many blood vessels have been cut across. Every embalmer I know would rather have a full autopsy than any partial dissection.

Every once in a while, especially in detective stories, a body must be exhumed for study. If the embalming has been really well done, a great deal can be learned from this delayed autopsy. Embalming fluid does a very good job of preserving tissues, and even years after burial, the autopsy of an embalmed body can yield excellent tissues for the preparation of microscopic slides. Embalming fluid consists principally of the same fixative material that the pathologist uses for the preservation of tissues from an immediate autopsy or from surgical specimens — a solution of formaldehyde gas in water, called formalin. Most embalming fluids are secret formulas, but it is no secret that most of them contain mostly formalin plus deodorants, color preservers, and other ingredients. Satisfactory tissues may be obtained from an exhumed body, whether previously autopsied or not, but of course, if there has been a previous autopsy, the viscera are not found in their usual logical arrangement. And naturally, bacteriological studies are not possible; embalming totally destroys bacteria, hence the good preservation. Studies of the killed and fixed bacteria preserved in the tissues can be carried out with special histological stains, but the result is not very complete or satisfactory.

It is well-known that embalming has a long and distinguished history. There is not a schoolchild who has not been told while studying Egyptian history, that the ancient pharaohs were embalmed after death. As mentioned in chapter two, the organs were placed in several jars, and embalming was carried out using various spices and resins; the entire body was desiccated with hydroscopic natron (sodium carbonate). The result was such satisfactory preservation that even microscopic studies can be carried out today, and many papers have been written on the diseases of the ancient Egyptians on the basis of actual autopsy of the mummies. Mummification, however, was not limited to the Egyptians. There are numerous examples of long-term preservation of human and animal bodies through freezing in ice, desiccation in desert sands, and burial in bogs, where the oxygen necessary for decay was excluded. These latter cases of mummification were apparently the result of chance rather than any deliberate efforts to preserve bodies, but even here, autopsies have provided a great deal of information about the diseases which were present in ancient and even prehistoric times.

Embalming is so generally practiced and accepted in the United States that many Americans do not realize that it is a relatively rare procedure throughout most of the world. Embalming was rare even in the United States until the 1860s, but the Civil War gave it a tremendous stimulus through the problem of returning bodies of battle casualties to their families for burial in their own family burial plots. This return of bodies is an ancient custom, but until the Civil War, had been limited to only the most important people. The common soldier was almost always buried or cremated locally. During the time of the Crusades, there arose a practice of boiling the body of a deceased knight to remove the flesh, so that the bones could be returned to lie in western Europe, but the Vatican took a dim view of this practice and it was stopped. I think that every English schoolboy knows that Lord Nelson's body was returned to England in a keg of rum after he was killed in the battle of Trafalgar. Other methods of preservation of bodies have included immersion in honey, coating with wax, and packing in salt.

Many of the bodies returned during and after the Civil War were so disfigured that the military authorities insisted that the casket not be opened by the relatives, so the family had to accept on faith that the corpse had been correctly identified, and there are on record numerous cases of soldiers returning after they presumably had been buried. One interesting case of a returned body was associated with the return of the deceased from General Adolphus Greely's ill-fated Arctic expedition of 1884. Bodies were returned only with the solemn promise from each family that the caskets would not be opened. It is the opinion of at least one family (and they said it in print) that the government wished to conceal the fact that the deceased had been eaten by the survivors — an understandable act that has been repeated often in humans under extreme conditions, but always an embarrassment.

So far as the records show, the American Civil War was the first occasion when there was a large-scale effort to return bodies, so embalming became an American practice at that time. In other countries, there is little objection to autopsies on the part of undertakers, since there is rarely any effort to embalm.

There is great variation in the attitude of funeral directors to autopsies, but generally most would prefer that the body not be autopsied. The reasons are obvious. Besides the difficulties already mentioned (delay, disfigurement, and damage to blood vessels resulting from an autopsy poorly done), there is an inevitable extra expenditure of time in preparation. The autopsied body takes at least thirty or forty minutes longer to prepare than the unautopsied, even in the best of embalmer's hands, and if examination of the brain has been included in the autopsy, another thirty to sixty minutes must be added. But the best and most ethical funeral directors will often assist the doctor in obtaining permission, if the relationship between the two professions are good in the particular community. Several times, I have been called by a funeral director to do an autopsy requested by the family, when the doctor who had treated the patient did not think an autopsy was necessary.

Other funeral directors, particularly those of the old school, may actively counsel the family to refuse autopsy permission, and this attitude is most common in communities where the pathologists have been less sensitive to the needs of the funeral directors. Some communities have such fierce competition between funeral homes that delay becomes an important factor, and autopsy may be discouraged by a funeral director who fears that the next-of-kin may change their minds about the choice of funeral home during the time it takes to perform the autopsy. The contract with the funeral director is not generally binding until the body is actually picked up for transportation to the funeral parlors.

There is one type of case where the funeral director will actively suggest that autopsy be done: the instance where cremation is desired, and there is an implanted cardiac pacemaker within the body. Pacemakers are becoming quite common, and the problem for the funeral director is growing. The problem is that some pacemakers, when exposed to the heat of cremation, will explode, and before this was well-known, a number of cremation ovens were extensively damaged by such explosions. Today, many funeral directors require that the person ordering his services sign a paragraph taking financial responsibility for any damage caused by an exploding pacemaker as part of the routine of cremation arrangements, whether or not it is known that there is a pacemaker in the body. Pacemakers today have an increasingly long period of service before they cease to function, and now have a lifetime of twelve to fifteen years, as opposed to the three-year replacement which was necessary only a few years ago. It is understandable that a family could forget that their deceased relative had had a pacemaker implanted, so the routine responsibility clause seems appropriate, and the smart undertaker will urge that autopsy be done, if only to remove a known pacemaker before cremation.

Pacemakers are implanted to correct a too-slow heartbeat or other rhythm problem, and the technique of implantation is not too complicated. Pacemakers are implanted by making an incision, most often in the anterior shoulder area, and dissecting to form a pocket under the anterior shoulder muscle (the pectoralis major). The pacemaker itself is placed in the pocket, and the insulated wire lead is slipped into the jugular vein nearby. The wire is then advanced, while watching by fluoroscope, down the jugular vein and the superior vena cava, to enter the right atrium of the heart, and onward into the right ventricle where it comes to rest with its uninsulated tip in contact with the heart muscle at the lower end of the ventricle. Then the pacemaker can stimulate the muscle by tiny bursts of electricity and cause the heart to beat at the regular rhythm of the electric shocks. Most pacemakers are made so they don't stimulate if the heart is beating at an acceptable rate, but send their little shocks only when the heart is not doing its job. They're ingenious, complicated, and expensive devices, and there are many people leading active lives today who would be either cardiac cripples or dead without this help. Pacemakers are powered by special, long-life batteries, formerly mercury batteries but today, more frequently, a lithium type, and it is the batteries which are the explosion problem in cremation.

There is another special problem for both doctor and undertaker with a particular type of pacemaker, which makes autopsy a necessity and practically a legal requirement, whether cremation or burial has been chosen. There has been developed a nuclear-powered pacemaker which, once implanted, should never need replacement because there are no batteries which can run down. But every patient eventually dies, and the Nuclear Regulatory Commission (NRC) requires that such pacemakers be removed from the body and returned to the commission. So autopsy permission must be given, if only to remove the pacemaker. And then there is a further problem for the doctor in these cases, because he is required to make a report to the NRC on the status of the patient every six months while he lives, and to accept responsibility for the return of the pacemaker when he dies. It's all very complicated, so it's not surprising that few of these nuclear-powered pacemakers have been used. The paperwork and the responsibility are discouraging, particularly now, when today's battery pacemakers will last fifteen years before they need replacement.

But, to return to the main discussion and summarize: it may be said that understanding and cooperation on the part of both of the valuable professions of pathologist and funeral director can advance the social purposes served by the autopsy, but all too often, this understanding and cooperation is lacking, and society suffers.

Addendum, included here because it doesn't fit anywhere else: in answer to many questions about gold teeth, the price of gold today makes some people "worth more dead than alive" because of extensive dental crowns and bridges. Is the funeral director permitted, upon the request of the next-of-kin, to remove such gold and return it to the family? The answer, as far as I have been able to determine, is yes. The pathologist may also perform this service for the family (although I never was asked to), but if he does, he would do well to see that the undertaker understands, so he won't be accused of stealing from the body.

CHAPTER TWELVE

THE AUTOPSY AND MEDICAL EDUCATION

In a way, it is to belabor the obvious to consider the impact of the autopsy on education. So much knowledge of anatomy and physiology has come from the autopsy in the past, and new knowledge is constantly being developed from the autopsy procedure today. Education is the imparting of knowledge — of facts, techniques, and philosophy — and that is what the autopsy is mostly about. I say "mostly" because the usefulness of the autopsy in medical-legal procedures and in public health disease control is well-established. But the service of the autopsy to education is far and away the most important aspect of its usefulness to society.

Education cannot be confined into multiple, small, restricted areas. It is a continuum across many disciplines. Thus the autopsy has been useful in basic biology, philosophy, and many other fields, but to no endeavor is it more important than to medical education. In truth, it is one of the most important procedures in the education of the doctor, because so much of the detailed knowledge which is necessary for the physician to possess is built upon the facts discovered at the autopsy table. Direct observation of the autopsy procedure is an essential for the understanding of the human body. It is true that, in recent years, physiology (the science of the complex quasi-chemical reactions in the living body) has outstripped anatomy in the development of new medical knowledge (although the electron microscope is beginning to reverse this), but without an understanding of the anatomy of the body, physiology becomes meaningless. The autopsy procedure is the backbone of medical education.

Medical education begins early, and continues throughout the lifetime of the conscientious physician. The basic attitudes, and some of the basic facts, are learned in junior high school general science classes, and even before that. High-school biology, chemistry, physics, and mathematics add to the structure, and college-level courses in these fields are part of the major labeled as pre-med. Of course, training in the humanities, in ethics and in philosophy are essential for the complete human being, and doctors need to be complete human beings, above all. But even at the college level, a great deal of direct knowledge of anatomy is taught. The dissection in comparative anatomy courses using fetal pigs, frogs, and other creatures is another step toward the understanding of human anatomy.

Upon entrance into medical school, the doctor-to-be gets a first taste of human anatomy. With the burgeoning of knowledge to be absorbed, the long hours spent in dissection of a human cadaver have been greatly curtailed in recent years, but the student today is still faced very early in medical school with the anatomy laboratory, and learns to dissect and learn from seeing and doing. He generally works as one of a team; most often, four students have one cadaver to dissect, and the procedure may take several months at a rate of three afternoons a week. The cadaver is the embalmed body of one who has died without a family to take care of burial, or more frequently today, the body of someone who has asked that his body be donated to the medical school. This is further discussed in chapter fifteen, on organ donation and body donation.

The embalmed cadaver leaves a great deal to be desired in giving the medical student a feeling for the nature of the tissues and organs of the body. The tissues are firmer than normal from the effect of the embalming fluid, and often, to aid the student, the arteries and veins have been filled with latex rubber material, colored red for the arteries and blue for the veins. The odor, while not unpleasant, is not like the odor of the living or recently living body. But the embalmed cadaver is the best we can do at this point, and soon the medical student will get his first chance to attend an actual autopsy at one of the hospitals associated with medical school. He has to be an observer, not a participant, but he begins to get an idea of what the autopsy is all about, and what the tissues of the human body are like.

One educational procedure which has not been widely instituted and which would seem to be valuable is the possibility of providing the beginning medical student with a clinical history of the cadaver which he must dissect in first-year anatomy. It is true that the major emphasis at this level should be normal anatomy, but it is my experience that no body is "normal" throughout. It strikes me that the whole experience of anatomic dissection would be even more educationally rewarding if the beginner could have a chance to relate items of clinical history to some of the variations caused by disease which are inevitably found in the body. Nobody dies without some disease, be it only generalized senile changes. Perhaps the reason that medical schools do not use this valuable instructional method is that it would be a nuisance to keep a clinical history along with every cadaver used, but one of the complaints about medical student attitudes is the callous impersonality with which he regards the cadaver he is dissecting. A clinical history might emphasize, if it does nothing else, that the body upon which he is working has been a living, breathing human being with joys and disappointments, and who has at last been relieved from suffering through death.

As medical training progresses, the chances to attend autopsies increase, and in some medical schools, the student gets a chance to become a real participant, to assist with the dissection, and to do a trial write-up of the autopsy he has been concerned with, complete with a discussion of the patient's clinical history, the apparent cause of death, and a presentation of all the gross and microscopic findings observed. He learns to observe and report, and organize his observations into a final diagnosis. It is an intellectually demanding exercise which will serve him well in later life.

By the time of graduation, the medical student should have learned to appreciate the value of the autopsy in his education, and as he progresses to his post-graduate training as a hospital resident physician, he gets a chance to follow cases from the hospital bed to the autopsy table. For the first time, the resident (they're all residents now; the "intern" is a thing of the past) has the direct responsibility (under supervision) for the care of the patient, and he begins to suffer the defeat of having a patient die in spite of all his efforts. Now he has a chance actually to see the heart valves and to correlate what he sees with the heart sounds he has been hearing through his stethoscope. He can get a chance to check the shadow-pictures called X-rays (or better, roentgenograms) with the actual appearance of the tissues themselves. At last, he can see the actual ravages of the disease which he has been fighting against, and which has defeated him. This is education at its best.

In certain disciplines of medicine, the hospital resident gets a chance to perform autopsies himself, as principal prosector. Obviously, the pathology resident performs autopsies as a primary duty. He learns not only the intellectual exercise of clinical-pathological correlation, but also must learn the complex techniques whereby information from the autopsy may best be demonstrated. Often, surgical training programs include a period of doing the day-to-day work of the pathology resident. It is particularly useful to the budding surgeon, because he gets a chance to touch unaltered tissue without the problem of bleeding, and he also gets an opportunity to practice some of the techniques of the surgical operation. Many times, I have seen the surgical resident on pathology service do a complete gallbladder removal before going on to the actual business of the autopsy itself.

At long last, the doctor completes his formal training. He has been through primary and secondary school, college, medical school, and four or five years of post-doctoral training as a hospital resident. Is he now "educated"? The answer to this has to be "yes and no." He now has sufficient education to undertake care of patients on his own responsibility, and thus to give back, in the form of care of the suffering, some of the tremendous investment society has made in training him for so long. But no one's education is ever finished; it is so very important for the physician to recognize this, and to continue the education process for all of the rest of his working life.

Generally speaking, doctors as a group are intelligent, dedicated, and socially useful people. In fact, in a lifetime connected with medicine from my earliest years as a child in a doctor's family to my recent retirement, I have known of very few doctors who could not be listed on the "plus" side of the ledger of humanity. But I do remember one doctor to whom I would not refer even the pet cat of my worst enemy. He had been graduated at the top of his class from an excellent medical school and great things were expected of him, but he had one outstanding defect: he thought that his education was complete and he never opened a book or journal, and he never attended an autopsy after graduating from medical school and starting practice. The result was that, after a few years in practice, he was totally out of date, and as the years went by, he fell further and further behind, until he became a real menace to society.

I tell this story to emphasize the importance of continuous education in medicine. Medical knowledge acquisition does not begin one September day when the first-year student enters the medical school doors, and cease four years later. Medical education begins years before medical school and continues for the lifetime of the physician.

The need for continuing education is evident in many fields, but nowhere is the need greater than in medicine. New techniques, new facts and new attitudes are continuously developing, and the doctor must work constantly to keep up. Most states of the United States now require formal continuing education credits as one prerequisite to renewal of the license to practice medicine, and the doctor's mail today is filled with flyers offering continuing education courses to fulfill this requirement. I regret to report that some of the courses offered are being treated more as a chance to take a tax-deductible vacation than as a real educational opportunity. But most courses offered are legitimate and useful and really act to prevent the sort of falling behind such as I've illustrated.

As I have said, the autopsy is the firm base upon which knowledge in other disciplines of medicine is built, but also the autopsy is directly concerned with the education of physicians at all levels. After all, every hospital has to be a teaching institution as well as a place to help patients get well, and perhaps the most significant duty of the pathologist is to be an educator. The autopsy room is primarily a classroom; the pathologist is a teacher; and the doctor is a student all of his life.

One of the most rewarding exercises in the continuing education of physicians — and the most fun — is the clinical-pathological conference, known to American physicians as the CPC. Why this technique of teaching has not been used more extensively in other countries I do not know, but for the past seventy-five years, the CPC has been one of the primary educational exercises of the American hospital — and it depends generally upon the autopsy to achieve its ends. A few cases may use findings at surgery instead of autopsy findings, but autopsy provides the necessary information for most of these exercises. The CPC is structured as follows: A case is selected where a patient has been studied and treated in the hospital, has died and been autopsied. A summary of the patient's course in the hospital is prepared, presenting in narrative style all the significant events of the patient's history: the physical examination, the laboratory findings, and the progress of the patient's disease up to the moment of death, but not giving any diagnosis. This summary is made available a week or more before the meeting where it will be presented, and a discusser who knows nothing of the actual case is chosen. At the meeting, the discusser is faced with the task of reviewing the case summary, and giving his reasoning that leads up to a diagnosis, working entirely from the case summary. After appropriate discussion, the physicians who actually treated the patient present the diagnosis they arrived at; and finally the pathologist who performed the autopsy presents the autopsy findings, and the diagnosis he has made on the basis of what he has observed.

Often there is agreement among all three principals at the CPC discussion, but sometimes there is wide disagreement. This is particularly true when the facts known before death are really misleading, taking the clinical staff toward a diagnosis which is not confirmed by the autopsy. The clinical summary can also mislead the discusser of the case, but it is regarded as unfair and a violation of the rules of the game to structure the summary deliberately to mislead the unfortunate discusser. The ideal case for a CPC is one which the clinicians did not diagnose correctly, but which can be diagnosed from the information available, and in which the autopsy findings clearly demonstrate the disease which should have been identified in life. Such cases are rare, but traditionally the pathologist is delighted to embarrass the clinicians — and get himself hated. Most cases are, of course, well-handled, but any interesting case provides a worthwhile educational experience.

The CPC developed from some case-teaching exercises used by Dr. Richard Cabot at the Massachusetts General Hospital in 1895, and by 1910 it had assumed virtually the current form. The procedure has been widely adopted throughout the United States and Canada, and is used mostly as a teaching device for staff physicians. It is sometimes used as a medical school exercise for those students who have completed at least some of their pathology training. Medical students are often required to study the case and hand in their own diagnoses before the discussion. I remember one student who always handed in the diagnosis of "subacute bacterial endocarditis" no matter what the clinical summary showed, because this disease is so variable in its manifestations and it masquerades as so many different diseases; this student reasoned, "I may be wrong most of the time, but when they give us a case of bacterial endocarditis — and they will, — I'll be the only one who gets it right!"

Every week for sixty years, the CPC meetings of the Massachusetts General Hospital or one of its associated hospitals have been published in the *New England Journal of Medicine*, that most prestigious of medical journals, complete with clinical summary, discussion, X-ray, laboratory findings, and the pathologist's findings from the autopsy. For many of these years, actual projection slides have been available for purchase by subscription, so that other hospitals can take the cases and discuss them as if they originated in their own hospital wards or rooms. Other published CPCs are available from organizations such as the College of American Pathologists.

The most rewarding exercises are those which are developed within the hospital itself, using cases treated by its own staff and discussed by its own staff. But the difficulty with this in the smaller hospitals of this country is the lack of enough cases to give a good selection, and the virtual impossibility of finding an interesting case that the selected discusser doesn't know about already. The news of interesting cases travels very quickly through the medical staff of any small hospital.

The CPC remains a fascinating game, played for real educational purposes by hospital staffs, and is often one of the high points of the education program of any hospital. It is, however, not the only educational use of the autopsy. The staffs of such clinical services as surgery, medicine, or other specialties meet regularly to discuss cases, and one prominent feature of such staff meetings is the review of deaths on the particular service. Death review is really rewarding from an educational point of view if autopsy has been performed, and a great deal is learned from the discussion of such cases.

The autopsy also serves in the education of paramedical professions. It is essential that nurses be exposed to the autopsy procedure, although I must say that they frequently avoid it. Not only nurses should attend autopsies, but also the technicians from the laboratory, the radiology department, and physical therapy. A good argument can also be made for using the autopsy in the training of orderlies and aides. Anyone who has a legitimate professional or occupational interest in viewing the autopsy should be admitted to the autopsy. Perhaps if more were done along these lines, there would be less of the unfortunate opposition to the autopsy procedure that is sometimes found among nurses and other hospital personnel.

Probably the most important contribution to education that autopsy can make is found through actual attendance at the autopsy table while the pathologist is performing both the dissection and the examination of the tissue slides through the microscope. The report of the autopsy presented to an audience in a meeting is of great value, but the opportunity to observe the procedure firsthand gives a reality to the case which cannot be equaled, no matter how many slides are projected and summaries of diagnoses are presented.

The whole question of education resulting from the autopsy inevitably blends over into the question of quality control, which will be discussed in the next chapter. After all, the educational value of learning through self-appraisal cannot be exaggerated, and quality control is essentially self-appraisal. The defeat of losing a patient to disease is hard on the doctor, but it would be worse if the doctor wasn't able to learn from the failure. The one best way to learn is through the performance of autopsy. If what might have been done better is discovered, then the next case of the same disease may not follow the same course. To say that "the doctor buries his mistakes" is a cruel charge, but there is some justification if he doesn't learn from each failure.

CHAPTER THIRTEEN

THE AUTOPSY AND QUALITY CONTROL

Routine autopsy of at least a sizable sample of all deaths is the single most important procedure in the quality control of medical care rendered to the public. This is generally recognized in the hospital setting, but by extension it can be said that autopsy can provide a mechanism for the assessment of the quality of medical care, whether within the hospital or not — and it must be admitted that quality control of medical care is sadly lacking outside the hospital.

In recent years, the careful review of the quality of any production of goods or services has become of greatest importance, and the techniques whereby quality is judged are many and various. Each batch of steel that is made is studied, every printing of postage stamps is subjected to sampling and review. The delivery of services, too, is carefully examined to see if it is up to established standards. The care of sick patients is basically the delivery of the service of health care, and must be reviewed to see if the patients are being treated according to the best therapy available.

Hospitals have a number of procedures whereby quality can be studied. The hospital laboratory runs samples of specially prepared material along with the specimens coming from patients, and the findings from these samples are compared for accuracy. The assay is generally unknown by the laboratory technicians doing the tests, and the results are analyzed by the laboratory director or may be sent away to a central facility where the findings are compared with those from other hospital laboratories which have analyzed the same material. There are extensive statistical tests which will give precise limits beyond which a specific laboratory test is significantly inaccurate. Other parts of the hospital have their own controls as well, such as the placing of vials of bacteria in the sterilizers to see if they are all killed.

To study the overall efficiency of medical care, medical audits have been instituted in many hospitals. Often, a committee will review, for example, the last fifty cases of a specific disease, examining the hospital charts for such things as the medication or surgery used, the length of hospitalization and the outcome, and comparing the results to those of other hospitals and to the standards published in books of medical therapeutics and surgery. Other techniques of medical audit include sampling a random selection of hospital charts irrespective of diagnosis to see if everything is in order. Has the doctor written an acceptable history? Has the physical examination as recorded been complete? Are the laboratory and X-ray studies ordered by the doctor sufficient or excessive? And so on. Such studies show how well each of the cases has been treated.

These procedures are retrospective, and occasionally medical audit committees will review the handling of cases actually in the hospital, and check their findings against those recorded by the attending physician. Medical audits are part of the peer review mechanisms which are being used increasingly in hospitals, often instituted by the hospital medical staff in order to be sure of giving the best care to patients, but increasingly required by state and federal authorities. Payment of an older patient's hospital bill by Medicare will not be made if the hospital does not have an appropriate quality assurance through the use of medical audits or other mechanisms.

Procedures for quality control are also instituted from outside the hospital by state and federal inspections, or by the voluntary reviews conducted by the Joint Commission for the Accreditation of Health Organizations. Perhaps the word *voluntary* should be in quotes, because the hospital is under great pressure to request the review of the J.C.A.H.O. because its reports are generally accepted as equivalent to inspection by the various government bodies, and the inspecting team tends to be less authoritarian and demanding than government inspectors are. The Joint Commission sends in a team of surveyors (a less threatening term than the word *inspectors*) consisting of a doctor, an administrator, a nurse, and a laboratory specialist to study the work and structure of the hospital. The laboratory specialist may not be sent if the laboratory has already been inspected and approved by the College of American Pathologists. The team may spend only one day at the hospital if it is small and uncomplicated, or a couple of weeks if it is large. They review everything, such as the structure of the board of trustees, the bylaws of the medical staff organization, the completeness of the hospital charts, the appropriateness of the modes of therapy offered, and all sorts of other questions related to patient care. The physical arrangements are not neglected, and fire hazards and other safety-related factors are examined in detail.

Internal review procedures, however, are even more rewarding. No one likes to be inspected by an outside agency, and hospitals have instituted other careful internal reviews. One of the most interesting is the tissue committee, which reviews the surgical cases, and here the pathologist is directly involved. In my own hospital, I studied every surgical procedure done in the operating room to assure that it was appropriate, and reported my findings to the tissue committee, a board of five doctors appointed by the president of the medical staff. The committee would hear my report, and select those cases about which it had any question for detailed review from the hospital chart. Certain types of cases were automatically reviewed; for instance, every case of operation for appendicitis which yielded a normal appendix was studied for justification of the operation. One should not be surprised that some appendectomies do result in the removal of a normal organ; if the history, the physical examination, and the laboratory results — or even any two of these three factors — are consistent with appendicitis, the surgeon must operate; a certain percentage of the time, the appendix will be normal and the symptoms due to some other disease. Of course, all the indications for operation must be carefully recorded on the hospital chart before the operation, so the reasoning that leads the surgeon to operate can be seen clearly. The tissue committee keeps a close eye on the percentage of normal findings in these cases, and if the surgeon is removing a normal appendix in twenty percent or more of his cases, he is either a poor diagnostician, or worse, he is operating in order to increase his income. But if the percentage of normals falls below seven or eight percent, I worry that the surgeon is waiting too long on questionable cases, and running the risk to the patient of a ruptured appendix and peritonitis.

Other typical operations which come up for detailed tissue committee review are surgery with a significant discrepancy between the preoperative and the postoperative diagnosis — hysterectomies with insufficient disease to justify removal, gallbladders without stones, operations which yield no tissue, and the like. Review of the entire patient's chart almost always shows such operations to be appropriate, but once in a while, a surgeon is revealed by the tissue committee procedure to be substandard, and is then disciplined by the medical staff executive committee, or may even be removed from the hospital staff entirely. I recall the case of one surgeon who had his privileges whittled down from no restrictions to a list of minor procedures, and finally had his authorization even to remove tonsils denied. I hate say it, but at the same time he was having all these surgical privileges restricted in our good hospital, he was continuing to do major procedures such as gastrectomy in a nearby second-rate hospital. And then he was caught stealing blood from the blood bank of our hospital to treat his patients in the poor hospital. I am pleased to report that he is no longer in practice of any kind. Cases such as this are, I'm glad to say, very rare in my experience. But this illustrates the need for the authority of groups like our tissue committee.

Once in a while these days, a doctor has to be restricted or removed from the hospital staff for alcoholism or drug addiction that affects his efficiency, but dishonest or really incompetent surgery of the type which is revealed by the tissue committee review is rare indeed. It wasn't too long ago, though, that a hospital with a very good reputation found when it started its own tissue committee that it was running an overall normal appendix rate of more than fifty percent. Such committees ensure against systematic problems like this. Most doctors are honest, hardworking, and genuinely interested in saving lives and in relieving suffering, and so these committees continue to function. And the occasional incompetent or venal physician is also revealed, and such revelation makes headlines in the newspapers, giving an erroneous impression that such doctors are more common than they actually are.

A few words must be said here about the "unnecessary operation" about which a few of our health planners are so vocal. I reject emphatically the concept that an appendectomy that yields a normal appendix should be assumed to be an unnecessary operation if the indications are present, as described above. How about hysterectomies, which are cited so often as unnecessary? It is quite true that many hysterectomies could be avoided, but at the cost of significant morbidity. Take the case of the woman who has constant uterine bleeding, producing an anemia which makes her feel so tired all the time that she can hardly accomplish each day's tasks. She's been given a trial of various medications without benefit. She could indeed drag along for years without operation, but I contend that such an operation is not unnecessary. It is needed to restore a quality of life which has been lost. Over and over, if one analyzes the list of unnecessaries cited case by case, one finds cases that are not necessary from the point of view of saving the patient's life, but are necessary to restore well-being. Perhaps I've been lucky in my medical staff associates, but in my experience, the truly unnecessary operation is rare indeed.

Useful as all the approaches to quality control in the hospital are, the best quality-control procedure is, as previously stated, the routine performance of autopsies. The findings in the autopsy room are unequivocal facts, and when compared with the diagnoses made by the clinicians who followed the particular case in life, they make clear in striking detail the accuracy and precision of those diagnoses. The physical examination of the living patient produces signs from which inferences may be drawn about the patient's diseases, but not too many actual facts.

One excellent physician I know refers facetiously to his stethoscope as his "guessing tube," and indeed the murmurs and wheezes he hears through the stethoscope are truly guesses — educated guesses which have been substantiated in similar cases over the years by the autopsy. But guesses they remain, and the ability to guess correctly is a real art, the art side of medicine, rather than the science. The accuracy of the physician's diagnoses can be judged ultimately by the autopsy procedure, and only by the autopsy procedure.

I have mentioned elsewhere that the vital statistics recorded by the various state health departments are terribly inaccurate and misleading. The doctor who makes out a death certificate is all too willing to put down a plausible but unsubstantiated diagnosis, or sometimes even an unlikely diagnosis if it will save some argument. Thus every case of chest pain which goes on to die is likely to be signed out as myocardial infarction or heart attack, in spite of the lack of any supporting evidence or any real investigation of other possible diseases. Autopsy is necessary as a quality control on the vital statistics records. Most investigators who work with public health statistics now decline to accept the listing of all deaths, and form their conclusions on autopsied cases only — which in itself introduces a statistical bias, but is found to be at least somewhat more accurate.

Of particular interest from a quality-control viewpoint are those cases where the attending physician has made out a death certificate expecting that an autopsy will not be done, and then through some chance an autopsy permission is obtained, and an autopsy is done. The result has shown a shocking discrepancy between the certified cause of death and the actual cause revealed by autopsy. The literature has many studies of diagnostic accuracy, and one of the most interesting is a study of deaths between 1917 and 1922 at a particular large hospital, where it was shown that there was a 32.6% incidence of unsuspected cancer in autopsied deaths. The study was repeated fifty years later, and in spite of all the boasted advances in diagnosis, and application of better and more precise methods, there was an incidence of unsuspected cancer in 26.2% of the deaths, and of incompletely diagnosed cases of cancer of 13.9%. This latter figure includes diagnosed cancers which were found not to be present when autopsy was done.

Another study which has recently been published, showed that, in 1,152 hospital autopsies representing 25% of the deaths within this particular large hospital, 39% of the main clinical diagnoses were not confirmed, and 66% of diagnoses of conditions contributing to death were not confirmed. The authors of this study demonstrated that accuracy of diagnosis did not improve with longer hospital stay, which should have given an opportunity to sharpen the diagnoses. They asked the clinical doctors to estimate how sure they were of the diagnoses, and they found that while there was a correlation between the clinician's confidence and his accuracy, 25% of the "fairly certain" diagnoses were wrong. The authors felt that this was an alarming situation, so they instituted a crash program of obtaining all the autopsies they could, and succeeded in getting permissions in 65% of the hospital deaths over a short period. Of the 154 cases studied, it was found that 15% of the clinical diagnoses were not confirmed, and 42% of the listed causes of death were not confirmed. The attending doctors felt that they were fairly certain of the diagnoses in 94% of the cases, but among those, 12% were not confirmed. In this second, shorter series, there were 44 cases which would not have been autopsied in the usual run of the 25% autopsy rate which was customary in that hospital, but had been obtained because of the intensive pressure of the study, and of these, 14% had diagnoses which were not confirmed, and 15% showed significant discrepancies. These earnest investigators point out, "The rapid proliferation of diagnostic modalities has led to a steady denigration of the autopsy as a learning and corrective exercise. So great is the confidence in the accuracy of clinical diagnosis that it borders on hubris. Nothing is foolproof, and … the autopsy, properly done, still remains the ultimate in quality assurance."

I find the statistics developed by these studies frightening. When applied to the very large number of unautopsied deaths within the hospital, and the larger number of deaths outside the hospital, the gross number of inaccurate diagnoses is appalling. So much of the information on which we plan the conduct of our public policy is inaccurate. If there was a system of routine autopsy of every death, in or out of the hospital, we would have a better understanding of what is killing out citizens, and could then make rational plans to improve the situation.

The autopsy also becomes an important tool in the quality control of medical-legal cases, as seen in chapter nine. Accuracy of diagnosis is indispensable in cases coming before a court for obvious reasons, and the quality of medical-legal work depends in very large measure on the autopsy procedure.

Without autopsy, the cause of death is always suspect and inconclusive. And without autopsy of at least a sizable sample of deaths, in and out of the hospital, any statistical conclusion regarding what our citizens are dying of is likely to be misleading. Autopsy is the ultimate test of the accuracy of diagnosis, and the results of autopsy may be used to reveal mistakes, whether they are applied individually to a specific physician, to the hospital as a whole, or to a geographic unit such as a state or nation. Without autopsy to illuminate the efficiency of medical diagnosis and care, the professions relating to health care are working in the dark, and society is poorly served.

CHAPTER FOURTEEN

SOME FAMOUS CASES – AUTOPSIED AND UNAUTOPSIED

The most memorable case of autopsy of a famous person in recent years is obviously that of the assassinated young president of the United States, John F. Kennedy. Here was a charming man, a consummate politician, and a scion of a wealthy family cut off in the prime of apparent health by rifle bullets. The shattered body, already clinically dead, was rushed to a hospital and officially pronounced dead after some of the usual maneuvers, designed mostly in this case to show that "everything that could be done" was done. Then the mistakes (or perhaps even deliberate mismanagement) began to occur.

The case was immediately taken over by federal authorities, and the local interest was completely ignored. By removing the body from local jurisdiction, the federal authorities committed a violation of Texas law for which there was no justification, and there is nothing in federal law which gave them the right to do so. The medical examiner of Dallas had the legal right and duty to perform the autopsy, and he was a pathologist with long experience in forensic pathology; his protests were ignored. Any legitimate federal interest could have been satisfied by allowing federal officers to assist the medical examiner. Instead, the body of the president was transported to Washington, and was examined by military pathologists who were not forensic experts. It is clear that some real experts should have been recruited, and knowing forensic pathologists as I do, I'm sure that many of them would have been delighted to come to the autopsy without pay. Forensic pathologists as a group are characterized by active egos and showmanship, and have never been known to shrink from the limelight.

The John Kennedy autopsy was a masterpiece of confusion, and it certainly appears to have been designed to conceal, rather than to reveal, the truth. The pathologists proceeded without informing themselves as to what had been done at the hospital as attempts at resuscitation. This is a basic mistake which led in itself to a serious misinterpretation regarding the anterior neck wound. There was no apparent effort to exclude inappropriate people from the autopsy room, and at least thirty people were allowed to be present. No pathologist can do a good job in the presence of such confusion. A medical corpsman was asked to take photographs, but then a Secret Service operative seized and destroyed the film. The military superiors of the pathologists clearly pressured them into a hurried investigation. Even the best of pathologists could hardly do a good job under such conditions. But the defects do not stop there.

The autopsy report, which I have examined, is a wilderness of deficiencies. The report is not dated, nor is the time of completion stated. Measurements from known body locations to the bullet wounds are not given, so their precise location cannot be determined. There is no description by which the paths taken by the bullets within the body can be traced. An underlying detail was ignored which had concerned the medical community for years (only as a point of interest, not relating to Kennedy's capacity to serve in the presidency). This was whether or not he had Addison's disease, an endocrine abnormality resulting from deprivation of the secretions of the adrenal gland. This condition is easily treated by supplementary endocrine medications, first described in 1849 by Thomas Addison, the brilliant English pathologist. There had been a likely suggestion that Kennedy's adrenals had been heavily damaged in the famous PT-boat sinking in the Pacific during World War II, and rumors of Addison's disease affecting the president had been around for a number of years. But the autopsy report does not mention the adrenal glands, diseased or normal! Indeed, none of the abdominal organs are described or weighed, an omission that not even a first-year pathology resident would make, and an essential feature of any complete medical-legal autopsy.

Perhaps the greatest defect of the autopsy report is the incomplete and inaccurate description of the bullet wounds, so that the angle of fire of the bullets that struck the president cannot be determined, and an accurate interpretation of the findings is therefore impossible. In spite of these inaccuracies, competent forensic experts have analyzed the material which is available and have concluded that the angle of fire reported to the Warren Commission was inaccurate, and that reinterpretation makes it highly likely that the wounds were caused by two guns, not one. All in all, one can be forgiven for suspecting that the inaccuracies of description were deliberately made for the purpose of concealment rather than clarification, since the bullet wounds were the primary disease for which the autopsy was done. The only likely conclusion is that the reports were deliberately fudged in order to conceal. Military medicine has rarely been marked by brilliance, but if this was stupidity, it exceeds even military stupidity.

The only way the entire situation makes sense is to postulate a conspiracy. I must add to the autopsy inadequacies a number of other investigations, such as the timing of the firing, which was too rapid to have come from one gun, and the deliberate removal of physical evidence at the scene of the murder (the details are too voluminous to be repeated here; they are readily available in the many books on this subject). If a conspiracy is postulated, all of the facts fall into a logical pattern. It would have to be a conspiracy at the very high levels of government. Such a conspiracy would explain the murder of Oswald by Ruby, the death of Officer Tippet (killed the same day, allegedly by Oswald), and all of the extreme pressure on the Warren Commission to bring in the report that it did. The whole story reminds one of the murder and replacement of Roman emperor.

In contrast to the autopsy on John Kennedy, the handling of the case of his brother, Robert is an absolute classic example of how the assassination of a public figure should be investigated. After the death by gunfire of this brilliant young politician, the members of the family, mindful of the sloppy or dishonest job done in the case of the president, earnestly cooperated with the local medical examiner in having the autopsy performed. The procedure was undertaken by Dr. Thomas Noguchi, one of America's leading forensic pathologists, who was assisted by two of his associates from the Medical Examiner Department of Los Angeles and three experts from the Armed Forces Institute of Pathology in Washington. A radiologist, and members of the surgical team who had treated Kennedy's neurosurgical problems between the shooting and his death were included. Appropriate photographers, police representatives, and secretarial and technical helpers were present, and a security guard systematically excluded all those who were not invited in by Dr. Noguchi. The autopsy started at 3:00 A.M. and continued for six hours and fifteen minutes, and hundreds of photographs were taken. The resulting report is precise and extensive; I have it at my elbow as I write this and it is most impressive. The clothing of the body is carefully described, including the damage caused by the attack. (This description is entirely lacking in the John Kennedy autopsy report.) Every detail is carefully described, and the course of each bullet wound is clearly identified. X-rays taken in the course of the autopsy are described in detail. And all the organs not actually damaged by the bullet trauma are included in the precise description. No questions have been raised about the quality of Dr. Noguchi's procedure. How much better it is to have such a report than the careless or perhaps deliberately botched investigation in the case of John Kennedy!

It is quite apparent that every jurisdiction should have a plan ready in case a prominent public figure is killed within its bounds. This is a simple matter of preparing for medical-legal emergency. It has been suggested that forensic pathology teams be ready at all times for such problems in the areas they serve, and be ready also to consult with nearby areas that do not have adequate personnel.

Not quite as bad as the botched autopsy is the non-autopsy in the death of the famous person where autopsy is clearly indicated. At least in these cases, there is more of a choice than just stupidity or unethical behavior. The case that comes to mind immediately is the sudden demise of Pope John Paul I, only ten days after his election. That there should have been an autopsy is obvious. Indeed, the death of any famous person should be investigated fully, in order to put down the rumors which will inevitably spring up no matter how clear the apparent cause of death. Papal autopsies are completely within the traditions of the Church. Pope Alexander was autopsied in 1410, and there have been many popes autopsied since.

In the death of Pope John Paul I, there were conflicting reports of the time and place of death, which suggests even more strongly that a full investigation with autopsy was needed, and the family of the pope demanded an autopsy. The Vatican authorities refused, and the body was buried. A large group of Catholic laymen in Rome and elsewhere believed, and still believe, that the pope's death was not due to natural causes, and they feel that Vatican refusal to have an autopsy indicates that the death was a conspiracy murder, and done by Vatican functionaries to remove a pope who was not to their taste. It wouldn't be the first time such a thing has happened.

Another death which should have been autopsied was that of Mary Jo Kopekne, the unfortunate young woman who was apparently a passenger in the car said to have been driven by Senator Edward Kennedy, which went off the bridge at Chappaquiddick Island. Please note the "apparently" and the "said to have" in the previous sentence. I've never been satisfied that the story given out was correct. The death was handled casually, and no autopsy was ordered. After all, many persons die in submerged cars and are certified as victims of drowning, without autopsy. The lesson here is the same as the previous case. Every death in which a prominent person is involved should be autopsied, if only to rule out a cause other than accident, which will inevitably be suggested in view of the public interest in the prominent person.

The sequence of events in the Kopekne death is interesting and instructive. The local medical examiner being away, the associate medical examiner was called to the scene. He was a general practitioner with a busy office practice who was well known as a conscientious physician in protecting the health of many residents of the island of Martha's Vineyard. The associate medical examiner job was a sideline for him, done as a public service to give needed coverage of the necessary absences of the medical examiner; doing the job probably cost him money, because the time spent on medical examiner work is very low pay compared to the remuneration from a busy practice. The first impulse of this busy doctor was to certify the death as a simple drowning, as he would in any similar case, but then he thought of the implications of the case and consulted the District Attorney, who assured him that there was no need for an autopsy from the legal point of view. Indeed, he actively opposed the procedure. There are great questions as to whether this opposition was the result of personal objection, or whether political pressure had already been brought to prevent the autopsy. Subsequent events suggest the latter, since there was a great deal of pressure against exhumation and autopsy of the body, and finally the courts ruled against exhumation, which left the matter in limbo.

The only things that seem sure, even today, about the Chappaquiddick accident is that an automobile with a young lady's body was found in the water. There were all sorts of rumors: was she indeed alive when the car went off the bridge, or had she been killed earlier and the accident faked to make the death appear to be a drowning? Were there two pocketbooks in the car, indicating that there was another female passenger who escaped? Was Senator Kennedy actually driving, or had he been drugged and the car driven off the bridge by someone else? With two brothers assassinated such a short time before, any "accident" which might befall Senator Kennedy would be suspect, and there are many who believe that this "accident" was actually an attempt on his life. He was supposed to drown when the auto went off the bridge, but his many years as a "Hyannis water rat" saved his life. An autopsy on the body of Mary Jo Kopekne would not have stilled all of the rumors, but it would have helped to squelch some.

Whenever a prominent person dies, there are bound to be rumors of foul play. One has only to remember the death of Adlai Stevenson, which occurred suddenly on the street in London, to recall rumors that he had been murdered much in the manner of the Bulgarian opposition leader who was killed on the streets of London by a sophisticated poison injected in his leg by a needle concealed in the tip of an umbrella. It took the exhumation and autopsy of the Bulgarian leader's body to prove the murder, after another unsuccessful attempt with the same weapon on another Bulgarian. Could not a similar device been used on Stevenson? Indeed, an autopsy would probably have confirmed the heart-attack story which was issued so suspiciously promptly after the death, but competent investigation would have prevented a lot of speculation.

While we're on the subject of famous persons and their manner of death where autopsy should have been done and wasn't, I must mention the case of Nelson Rockefeller. He died under rather embarrassing circumstances in the apartment of a female acquaintance, and while there was no indication of foul play and it seems likely that the cause was a heart attack while engaged in strenuous physical activity, an autopsy should have been done. It was not done, apparently because of pressure from the family, to which the chief medical examiner of New York acquiesced. I doubt if the results of the autopsy could have been any more embarrassing, and might have been less so than the rumors which were circulated. Incidentally, the chief medical examiner was fired soon afterwards, not for dereliction of duty, but apparently for hinting about the possibility of some of the rumors having been true. It would have been better if he had been dismissed for insisting on an autopsy over family opposition.

It should be remembered that we are not that much different from the people of the Roman Empire, where many emperors and others were poisoned, smothered, or otherwise done away with, and the public given to understand that the cause was a natural death. In an atmosphere of secrecy and intrigue fostered by agencies such as the Central Intelligence Agency or the Federal Bureau of Investigation, it is not surprising that rumors of secret murders exist, and in many cases seem probable. One has only to think of the death of Karen Silkwood, who was killed in an "automobile accident" after she opened the question of nuclear poisoning of workers at the Kerr-McGee nuclear plant in Oklahoma. It seems most likely that she was deliberately murdered, yet no firm proof has been demonstrated, and no autopsy was done.

One of the most interesting cases of death of a famous person, with autopsy being done, was that of Eleanor Roosevelt. She was an energetic woman who was carrying a schedule that would exhaust anyone half her age, but in 1960, she developed symptoms of fatigue and malaise. After studies were performed, it was first thought that she was suffering from leukemia. Further study led to a diagnosis of aplastic anemia, so she was treated with cortisone, which has been effective in some cases of this disease. She was never really well again, and by the summer of 1962, she had to be hospitalized. She developed fevers, sometimes reaching a level of 105° F, and continued to deteriorate. Finally, only two weeks before her death, the right diagnosis was made. She was suffering from generalized tuberculosis, which had largely replaced the bone marrow and caused the anemia by destroying the blood-cell-forming tissues of the marrow. This diagnosis was confirmed by the autopsy. In retrospect, there are several questions raised by this case. Cortisone treatment is just the wrong thing to do in cases of tuberculosis because it blocks some of the body's natural mechanisms that combat infection and inflammation. Mrs. Roosevelt had X-ray evidence of old tuberculosis from an infection many years before, and no case of tuberculosis should be regarded as cured, only arrested. Another possibility is that she became infected by contact with her doctor, to whom she was closely attached, and who had had to undergo sanitarium treatment of that disease in 1947. In any case, the autopsy proved that Mrs. Roosevelt died of miliary (so-called because the widespread lesions are thought to resemble millet seeds) tuberculosis, and her death was hastened by the cortisone treatment she received.

When Albert Einstein died in 1955, his body was autopsied at the hospital in Princeton, N.J. He had been having increasing back pain and malaise, and it was suspected that arteriosclerosis had so damaged his arteries that the aorta had begun to form an aneurysm, or potential blowout, with some early leakage of blood. He was much opposed to the idea of operation, which could have replaced the affected area with an artificial fabric blood vessel made of nylon or other material. The results of such operations were not, in those days, as highly successful as they are today. In any case, Einstein grew worse and died. In accordance with his wishes the autopsy was not published, but it was stated that the autopsy confirmed the diagnosis of aneurysm. His body was cremated and the ashes scattered at an undisclosed location, but the brain, which had so shaken the mathematical and physical sciences over the many years of its activity and contributed so much to the world's knowledge, was placed in formalin solution to harden for later examination. It seems, though, that no one wanted to take the responsibility for sectioning the brain, so it remained in formalin for years, being moved from one hospital laboratory to another as pathologists moved around. I understand that it has now been examined, at least partially, and it shows no anatomic difference from the brains of the most mundane and routine humans who come to autopsy, which was to have been expected, since intellect is not a function of any known anatomic variation.

In considering the history of the autopsy, it is interesting to know that, two hundred years before the definitive work of Rudolf Virchow, who more than anyone else was responsible for making the autopsy the precise procedure it is today, the autopsy was well-established in northern Europe, as is made evident by the autopsy on the body of Ludwig van Beethoven. This musical genius died following a strenuous altercation with his brother Johann, which made him so angry that he rode back to Berlin in an open carriage in bad weather in December. He became ill, not surprisingly, and deteriorated gradually over the next three months, with apparent pneumonia complicated by congestive heart failure. After his death, which occurred characteristically in the middle of a furious hail and thunderstorm, the first move was to make the famous death mask, and then Dr. Johann Wagner proceeded with the autopsy. Of particular interest was the brain and the auditory nerves, in view of his progressive deafness. The following is quoted from a translation of the autopsy report: "The auditory nerves were shrunken and indistinguishable; the auditory arteries that paralleled them were thickened and cartilaginous as though stretched over a raven's quill. The left, much thinner auditory nerve, originated in three very thin grey fibrils, and the right nerve in a single, thicker pure white strand, both arising from the substance of the fourth ventricle, which in this area was of a firmer consistency and more vascular. The convolutions of the brain, ordinarily much softer and edematous, here appeared twice as deep and more numerous than usual. The cranial vault was of a great thickness throughout, and approximately a half-inch thick."

So it is clear there was a good anatomic explanation of his deafness, due to sclerosis of the blood supply to the auditory nerves, which subsequently degenerated. An interesting incidental finding was the thickening of the skull, which can be interpreted as probable Paget's disease of the bone.

Another musician who died and came to autopsy was George Gershwin. This brilliant young artist was his usual exuberant self until February of 1937, when he had a blackout preceded by a sense of smelling burnt rubber while he was conducting a concert in Los Angeles. He recovered quickly, and most of the audience didn't notice the lapse. By four months later, however, he was having increasing headaches and dizziness, and finally was diagnosed as having a probable brain tumor. Brilliant neurosurgeons were called, but they were on the East Coast, and his condition was so bad that they advised immediate operation by local surgeons. A tumor was found and partially removed from the right temporal lobe of the brain, but the patient died within hours. Autopsy confirmed that a very rapidly growing brain tumor was present and was incompletely removed. Indeed, it was so extensive that it could not have been removed completely.

This is just a sampling of autopsy and non-autopsy cases involving a few famous people. Many more cases could be cited, which would illustrate further some of the importance of the performance of autopsy, and some of the uses to which the procedure can be put. And I particularly wish to emphasize the necessity of autopsy in every case involving a famous person, about whom rumors may arise.

CHAPTER FIFTEEN

BODY DONATION — ORGAN DONATION

In recent years, there has been a marked growth of interest in anatomic gifts, i.e., the donation of organs for transplantation and research, and the donation of intact and unautopsied bodies to medical schools for the purpose of furthering medical education. Body donation has been with us to a limited extent for many years, but organ donation is a more recent development, a result of the tremendous advances in surgical technology which makes organ transplantation a legitimate therapy for certain diseases. Recently, many states have recognized the appropriateness of anatomic gifts to the extent of including in the automobile driver's license application the opportunity to indicate the desire to make such a gift, and placing that information on the license itself.

The donation of the body to the medical school has a direct effect on the principle of performance of autopsy in every possible case, for obvious reasons. If the body is to be made available for medical school dissection, it cannot be available for autopsy. The social usefulness of advancing medical education must be balanced against the purpose served by autopsy used to understand disease and its trends in society. Occasionally it becomes a difficult matter for next-of-kin to judge which procedure will benefit the community more. Generally however, when medical schools need cadavers, the use of the body to further the training of doctors-to-be will be of equal importance in the long run to the benefits to be derived from the understanding of disease by doctors already in practice. When there is a real question as to the cause of death, or when there is a rare and difficult disease at hand, the need for autopsy supersedes the need for a cadaver for medical school dissection. Most deaths occur following diseases which are not a puzzle to the attending physicians, and while some of the benefits to the family and to medical knowledge may be lost, the need for cadavers for anatomic dissection is usually very great, and medical students must have cadavers for their training.

Body donation used to be possible only through a decision of the next-of-kin made after the patient had died. Similar to the situation regarding autopsy permission noted in chapter six, the courts used to hold, regarding body donation, that any permit signed or decision made before the actual death was invalid, on the basis that those giving permission were not in possession of all the facts (medical, emotional, or otherwise) that would permit them to make an informed decision. I'm glad to say that this restrictive ruling has been changed in most states by the passage of anatomical gifts laws by the various legislatures. Now the person himself is legally permitted to make the decision as to what is to be done with his body. He may select either donation of the entire body, or donation of specific organs on his own responsibility. If no election is made, then the next-of-kin may still make choices after the patient expires, and most hospitals and physicians wisely prefer to get the signatures of the next-of-kin, confirming the choice of the deceased in any case, in order to prevent future repercussions and accusations which, although having no legal effect, are nevertheless annoying and embarrassing.

In the past, and still to a large degree today, bodies are obtained from state and municipal hospitals in cases where there is no next-of-kin or other claimant for the body. This source of cadavers for dissection is largely drying up because of the increased numbers of persons who have at least burial insurance, or are buried by government through veterans programs or other similar arrangements. The number of completely indigent persons without survivors or access to any program which will bury them is small and growing smaller, year by year, so it is evident that, with larger numbers of medical students to be trained, the need for body donation by people of good will is increasing rapidly.

If body donation is elected, the procedure is quite simple. The anatomy department of the medical school in the locality is notified within a few hours after the death; if death is in a hospital the hospital officials will generally take care of this, so no further activity is required of the survivors. The medical school will arrange transportation, generally using the services of a local undertaker, and will assume all costs from the time of notification. The body is taken to the anatomy laboratories of the medical school and carefully embalmed. The body is carefully wrapped to prevent dehydration, and placed in a cool room where it will be held for months or even a year, pending the start of the next sessions of the anatomy class.

Most medical schools assign four students to each cadaver, but sometimes a shortage of bodies leads to the assignment of six or even eight students. When four students are assigned, they are divided into two teams of two each, and since a large number of the body structures are paired, each team has the opportunity to see and do everything required. Traditionally, the leg and arm are dissected first, with the medical students learning and increasing their skill at dissection so that when the finer structures are approached, their skills will be adequate for the problems encountered. The muscles are identified, the blood vessels are traced, and the nerve distribution dissected and identified. The bony structures are generally studied not from the cadaver, but using a skeleton, and these are becoming increasingly hard to find; most of them come from southeast Asia, and they are becoming very expensive. Excellent skeletons are now becoming available that use plastic reproductions rather than actual bone — but these are even more expensive.

Lectures are held all through the semester while the students are studying anatomy, with subject matter appropriate to the area being dissected at the time. The anatomy of the abdominal and thoracic organs is then undertaken, and finally the head and neck structures are studied. The brain itself is generally so poorly preserved in the embalming process that brains obtained from autopsies are generally used for the central nervous system anatomic dissection.

After the study of the body is complete, and this may be several months later at the rate of two or three long afternoons at the dissecting table each week, all parts of the body are returned to the specific casket which has been assigned to the particular cadaver, and the caskets are transferred to a cemetery. My own experience is with a cemetery owned and operated jointly by all the medical schools in the area. Some other medical centers have facilities for cremation, which may be elected by the family when the donation papers are first made out. Of course, the family may claim the casket and bury it in a family plot at their own expense if they wish, or arrange for cremation on their own. But if burial by the medical school is elected, appropriate services are held at the cemetery to which the family of the deceased is invited, and the procedure of body donation is completed.

My own mother-in-law chose body donation and she used to tell her grandson that she "was going to medical school." He knew she had not been to college, so how was she going to medical school? It was a longtime family joke, and when she died of Guillain-Barré syndrome following immunization for influenza at age eighty-nine, she indeed went to medical school. About eighteen months later, we were notified that the body was ready for burial — and she had chosen to be buried in the medical school cemetery. We went to the services, which were deeply moving and most satisfactory. Separate services were held for Jewish, Catholic, and Protestant bodies. About thirty-five bodies donated to medical school were buried in the service we attended, each in a separate, identified grave, and with a number of relatives in attendance. Later we had a memorial concert at the nursing home where she died, so her friends could attend.

The advantage to the family of electing body donation is very real, beyond the desire to aid medical science. Not only is there a highly significant contribution made to advance medical education, but there is an excellent financial saving, which may be very useful to the family in view of the many monetary demands which fall on the survivors following the death of a relative. The medical school assumes all of the costs of handling the situation, from transportation of the body, embalming, furnishing the casket, burial, and finally the funeral service. This may be a highly significant saving to a family, because the costs of these things, even at the absolutely lowest-cost choices, will run to eight or nine hundred dollars today in most areas, and may be expected to increase in the future, with some parts of this country having considerably higher costs. It's not just that I am a stingy Yankee that I have elected body donation for myself. I must admit that the financial saving interests me, but I do want to make an appropriate contribution to medical education.

Organ donation, on the other hand, does not interfere with a meaningful autopsy procedure. Indeed, it almost requires autopsy, and most organ donation cases come to full autopsy examination. Some jurisdictions even require an autopsy permit for organ donation, since it is a procedure on a dead body, and if a full autopsy is not to be done, then the autopsy permission must be specifically restricted to the one procedure of organ removal. I have, on occasion, received a permission slip with the restriction, "Limited to the removal of eyes for Eye Bank," in which case I did just that and sent the body to the undertaker.

The greatest problem with organ donation is the matter of obtaining the particular organ in a viable condition; it would do no good to transplant an organ which was dead and could not function. For most organs, this means that the body has to be maintained by life-support systems in a quasi-living condition up to the moment of the removal of the organ or organs. The commonest situation in which organ removal for transplantation is possible is the case of brain death in which respiration, and sometimes heart action, is maintained artificially. It is not too difficult to maintain respiration by machine. The anesthesiologist is very familiar with "bagging" a patient, that is, breathing for the patient by squeezing by hand a large rubber bag attached to a mask over the patient's nose and mouth. And there are a number of machines which similarly maintain breathing without manual manipulation of a bag.

Maintaining heart action is somewhat more complicated. External cardiac massage may be used for two or three hours, but then even the hardiest emergency medical technician becomes weary. An electric wire may be inserted into a vein and pushed along the course of the veins to carry the tip of the wire into the right ventricle of the heart. The wire is then connected to a pacemaker, which sends tiny electric shocks to the heart to stimulate it to beat regularly.

With the body kept "alive" by these life-support machines, the organ donation procedure can go forward, if there is no hope for real life or recovery of the patient. This creates a problem for doctors, lawyers, clergy, and the public at large: when is the patient dead? The matter is still under active consideration in many quarters, but it seems now to be coming down to a question of whether the brain is alive or not. Therefore, the next move in an organ donation case, after the matter of both respiration and heart-action maintenance, is to check the brain. Tiny electrodes are placed at several locations on the scalp, and are attached to a multi-channel recording device which records the electrical activity of the brain. Every truly living person has electric activity arising from the function of the central nervous system nerve cells, and this activity can be recorded on paper. This is popularly known as brain-wave recording. The brain is active electrically even during deep sleep if it is alive, so the recordings of this electroencephalograph machine can really define whether or not the patient is alive. If the recordings show only straight lines with no wave activity, then the brain is dead; and if the brain is dead, no matter what the heart and lungs, or the muscles and vessels or other portions of the body are doing, the patient is dead.

The removal of organs for transplantation may then proceed, and as promptly as possible, using careful surgical technique so that the removed organs will not become contaminated and carry disease to the recipient. The first major organ used for transplantation, excluding blood for transfusion and corneal transplants, was the kidney. The kidney transplant program opened at the Peter Bent Brigham Hospital in Boston, and it utilized, not the kidneys of a person who had died, but for this first experimental program, one of the kidneys of a living person whose identical twin needed a transplanted kidney to replace the function of his kidneys which had failed. The use of an identical twin was then necessary to get around the problem of tissue rejection. To say that no two people are alike is correct, except in the case of the immune systems of a pair of identical twins, whose immune antigens are just as identical as the shapes of their noses. The human body recognizes as foreign any tissue or organ from another person, except a transplant from an identical twin. Fraternal twins are another matter; they may be quite different in their immune systems. The Brigham hospital statisticians calculated that there would probably be only seven cases in the world with sufficient disease to require the kidney transplant operation who also would have an identical twin with two healthy kidneys, one of which could be removed. Within a couple of years, seven such cases were found and operated successfully, and then there were no more to be found — a triumph for statistics!

With the techniques of the surgery of kidney transplantation well worked out, surgeons in Boston and elsewhere proceeded to transplant from the living, using at first cases of close family relationship, which would likely be somewhat similar in antigenic makeup to the proposed recipient, but it was found that the transplanted organs were nearly all destroyed by rejection fairly promptly unless immunosuppressive medication were given to the recipient. Immunosuppression results in the patient's immune systems not recognizing as foreign the transplanted tissues. This is very useful for transplantation, but it destroys the body's ability to fight off foreign invading bacteria which cause a number of diseases. However, with antibiotics and other means, medical science has now learned how to walk the narrow path between organ rejection on one hand, and overwhelming disease on the other. This makes possible the use of kidneys from unrelated individuals and the transplantation from the bodies of very recently dead organ donors. The procedure is no longer experimental, and is a well-established mode of therapy which has prolonged the lives of many patients with kidney failure. A great deal has now been learned about compatibility of tissues, and HLA matching has greatly improved the acceptance of a transplanted organ.

The criticism has been voiced in many quarters concerning

the removal of kidneys from living donors, no matter how willing and enthusiastic they may be. In too many cases, the transplanted kidney went on to develop the same disease that destroyed the recipient's previous two organs, the recipient hadn't really been helped, and the donor was left with only one remaining kidney. Some people are born with only one kidney, and this situation is completely compatible with life as long as nothing untoward happens to the single organ, but those of us who have been endowed with two kidneys are much safer, in case accident or disease damages one of our two. Is it justifiable to create a one-kidney situation in a healthy donor? It's a difficult point, and today, most kidney transplants are done as a result of organ donation from recently deceased persons.

Other organ donation programs are now becoming accepted. The dramatic operation of heart transplant is a surgical tour de force, and is becoming established as really legitimate therapy. It is a wonderful thing that surgery has advanced to such a point that heart transplant can be done and there are some patients who have had significant prolongation of life from the procedure, but the expense is astronomical and a similar amount of money and effort could save so many more lives in other cases. In any case, heart transplant may soon be replaced by the implantation of a mechanical pump. This emphasizes that in many ways, the heart is the simplest and most unsophisticated organ of the body. All it does is pump, and the outlook for a successful, mechanical, implantable machine is good indeed.

Still experimental is the liver transplant. It has been tried, often unsuccessfully, in cases of liver failure, generally where the liver of the recipient is expected to resume functioning in a short while, so that the transplanted organ may be removed. Even the use of pig liver has been tried for this purely temporary purpose. The use of a mechanical device to do the work of the liver should be considered. I once asked a liver specialist if this were possible, and he said yes, but in view of the many different functions of the liver, it would have to be the size of a house trailer. Heart-and-lung transplants have been tried, successfully, but no one to my knowledge has tried a transplant of the pancreas, or any other organ. Spleen transplant would make no sense, since the spleen is unnecessary for continued life, and thyroid is very easily replaced by just giving thyroid medication by mouth.

I know of only one attempt at adrenal transplantation, years ago, and it gave such promise of success that I cannot understand why it hasn't since been done. A young man with Addison's disease, which is the result of the destruction of the function of the adrenal gland, had embryo adrenal tissue transplanted into a convenient location in his anterior abdominal wall. Within months, his symptoms of Addison's disease cleared up, and a small mass was now palpable in the area of the transplant. Apparently embryo tissue is much less likely to be rejected by the recipient's immune system, for the principles of immunosuppression were not known at the time. In any case, in order to document the success of the procedure, a surgeon was persuaded to take a small biopsy of the mass to prove that it was now adult-type, functioning adrenal tissue. But the surgeon was apparently not fully instructed as to what was wanted, and he proceeded to remove the whole mass, so the patient went on to die of Addison's disease a number of months later. The mass removed, seen under the microscope, was indeed adult-type adrenal tissue.

Eye donation, or rather cornea donation, is quite another matter from the donation of internal organs. Here the donor does not need to be kept in a semi-alive state until the organ is removed. The eyes used for cornea transplant may be removed even five or six hours after death, and so may be done by the pathologist in the autopsy room, if sterile precautions have been maintained. The whole eye is easily removed by cutting the attachments of the six muscles that move the eye and the optic nerve, and the eye is placed on a sterile, saline-soaked gauze pad in a sterile jar, with the cornea facing up. The moisture from the gauze vaporizes to keep the cornea from drying out if the jar is tightly sealed, and the eye may be transported several hundred miles to a facility where the cornea can be removed and sewed in placed of the damaged cornea of a recipient. Immune rejection is not a problem because the cornea is so poorly supplied with blood that immune antibodies do not reach it in sufficient quantity to do any harm.

Skin transplants have not worked out except as a temporary covering for burned areas; rejection occurs in every case, except identical twins, and new artificial skin preparations are becoming available for cases with large skin-denuded areas, so that this type of transplant is disappearing.

Appeals are frequently received from the Temporal Bone Bank people. Here the donor tissue is not used for transplant, but for research which it is hoped may give some aid to the prevention and treatment of deafness and other ear diseases. The donor's family may be deprived in these cases of the emotional satisfaction of visualizing a portion of the deceased living on, and thus achieving a sort of immortality, but the procedure is very valuable and may do even more good than some of the organ transplant attempts. For a number of years, pathologists have been, without specific organ-donation permission, removing the pituitary glands of autopsied bodies and delivering them to the National Pituitary Agency, which extracts the growth hormone used to treat the lack of this hormone and consequent dwarfism (achondroplasia) where it occurs. New genetic engineering has made it possible for other forms of life (bacteria especially) to produce *human* growth hormone so this form of donation may soon be unnecessary.

I think that it should be remembered that one form of organ transplant is very common indeed and has been practiced for many years. It does not involve a deceased donor, and it causes no disability to a living donor. I am speaking of blood transfusion, which is well established as legitimate therapy today. Cadaver blood has been used to a limited extent in the Soviet Union, but in general, the use of living volunteer donors has proved to be most successful. Immune rejection by the recipient occurs only when the blood has not been correctly matched for the few antigen-antibody reactions that occur with blood cells, so the use of identical twins is not necessary. With organ transplant, similar attempts are made to cross-match, but the practically infinite number of antigens present make this practically impossible. With blood, there is only the A-B system, and the Rh system to cross-match in most cases, so immunosuppression is not needed. Blood donation is well established and unlikely to be replaced, although there are attempts to manufacture artificial blood so that donation will be unnecessary.

After the removal of organs for transplant donation, there is nothing to preclude the completion of a thorough autopsy examination. Indeed, it would seem wise to know as much as possible about the disease systems of the deceased, if only to help in the specific case of the recipient of the organs transplanted. There is a legitimate question as to what diseases might have been transplanted along with the organs, and AIDS has become a real problem in this connection. If there is evidence of liver disease in the donor's body, there might be a likelihood of hepatitis in the recipient, and the physician would like to know about it so he could head off the disease. Autopsy is really most necessary for transplants except in the case of cornea, and even here a history of AIDS, liver disease, or syphilis will lead to the refusal to use the cornea for transplant purposes.

Organ donation, on the other hand, does make the body unacceptable for whole-body donation to medical schools for education purposes, again with the exception of eye-bank donation which is perfectly acceptable. So the well-motivated individual faced with a decision between organ donation or body donation, or the family of a deceased or brain-dead patient has to make choices, and will probably be wise to talk to physicians, clergy, and others about the appropriate action in a particular case. What will serve humanity best, organ donation and a subsequent autopsy, or body donation for educational purposes? The nature of the deceased's disease may make quite a difference, but often it will be a difficult choice.

CHAPTER SIXTEEN

PAYING FOR THE AUTOPSY

It is clear that autopsy is an expensive procedure, utilizing as it does the services of a highly trained physician, a diener, an histologist, and a typist at the minimum, and requiring equipment and supplies, and an area generally exclusively dedicated to the procedure, the autopsy room. Heat, light, and water must be supplied, and the services of a large troop of support personnel, such as maintenance engineers, sweepers, aides, file clerks, and others, contribute to the successful completion of the autopsy. But the bulk of autopsies in the United States, and all over the world, are performed with no fee being charged. Very few hospital autopsies are billed to the family of the deceased, and medical-legal autopsies are paid for by appropriate government agencies at far below their actual cost. How is this miracle wrought?

To calculate the cost of the autopsy, it is an obvious procedure to add up all the expenses connected with autopsy performance over a year, and divide the sum by the number of autopsies performed. This has been done with greater or lesser accuracy by pathologists and hospital administrators many times over, and when all the costs are totalled and apportioned to the individual autopsy, the figure stands today at well over three thousand dollars, and it continues to rise, year after year, with inflation.

Setting aside an adequate space for autopsies, and providing heat, light, and water to the area is expensive for the hospital; and the area is then not useful for anything else because it is appropriately regarded as a contaminated area. New hospital construction rarely provides for a new autopsy room, and the dingiest corner of the basement of the oldest building of the hospital is generally where the autopsy room is found. Architects and administrators generally see it as a nonincome-producing area and thus give it little consideration, but the equipping of the autopsy room is expensive; an adequate autopsy table of stainless steel, with running water and electric service costs a great deal, although I know of at least two cases where the pathologist had his table made out of old marble slabs from a shower stall that was being removed. The instruments the pathologist uses represent a considerable investment — although some hospitals save money by supplying the autopsy service with discards from the operating rooms for some of the instruments required.

Certain costs are assignable only partially to the cost of the postmortem. For instance, the morgue refrigerator is used for most of the hospital deaths, regardless of whether the body is autopsied or not. The processing of the tissue samples taken at autopsy is performed by the same histology technical staff, using the same equipment, who process the tissue specimens which come to the laboratory as a result of the removal of organs or tissues in the operating rooms of the hospital. The typist who transcribes the pathologist's dictation is occupied only part of the time with autopsy work in the average hospital. And the record-keepers who file the autopsy reports are generally the ones who handle the charts of all the patients in the hospital. The salary or other remuneration of the pathologist himself is only partially assignable to the costs of the autopsy.

All of these factors are considered, and under the most careful cost analysis, the cost of the average autopsy today (this is written in 1992) lies somewhere between $3,000 and $3,500. Of course, if a hospital maintains all the equipment and personnel for a complete autopsy service, but does only one or two autopsies per year, the cost will be astronomical.

The hospital generally handles the costs of autopsy by regarding it as part of the hospital overhead, and with considerable justification. The hospital is required, if it is to receive the approval of the Joint Commission for the Accreditation of Health

Organizations, to provide the service. This organization was formed to assure that hospitals are adequate for their purposes by the American College of Surgeons, the American College of Physicians, the American Medical Association, and the American Hospital Association; it states as one of its standards, "Space, equipment, and personnel shall be available for a necropsy service that is adequate for the needs of the hospital. Each necropsy shall be performed by a pathologist or a physician who is sufficiently qualified in anatomic pathology."

If the hospital does not meet this standard, or any of the other stringent standards of the agency, it will not be accredited by the Joint Commission, and in many cases will be unable to survive financially or medically because people will not use its services. While the Joint Commission is not an official government agency, many of the official agencies utilize its inspections and approvals as evidence that the hospital is eligible to receive payments under various programs of government assistance, without which it could not survive. Approval for payments under the Medicare program requires J.C.A.H.O. approval, or an inspection by an official agency which is just as stringent as this voluntary agency. The same standards are used and applied in the same way, so most hospitals elect to go through the survey of the Joint Commission, and meet its standards.

We see, therefore, that it is not a miracle that autopsies can be financed. The costs are just added into the general overhead of the hospital and handled in much the same way as the costs of heating, maintenance, and all the other routine costs of operating a hospital. If the pathologist is salaried by the hospital, his salary is similarly absorbed, and if he is paid by the case, this cost goes into overhead.

There is further justification for handling the costs in this way: the autopsy, as previously explained, is a necessary part of the general education program of the medical staff. And, as shown in another chapter, it is an important factor in quality control of the efficiency of the medical care offered by the hospital; quality control costs are universally accepted as a legitimate part of overhead.

One of the controversies which plague the profession of

pathology, however, is the question of what particular fund pays for the pathologist's services when the costs are assigned under Medicare. The Medicare B Trust Fund does not pay for them at the time that this is written, because it says that the autopsy is not a service to a patient; the pathologist feels that the autopsy is a professional service and should be paid in the same manner as other professional remuneration. Hopefully this question will be resolved by the time the reader encounters this paragraph.

In one sense, the autopsy is very inexpensive. Once the equipment is all in place and no extra personnel have to be hired, then the cost is very low indeed. In other words, in a hospital that does four hundred autopsies a year, what is the added cost if one more autopsy is performed? Suppose the pathologist would only be sitting and reading, that the diener would be "goofing off," that the histologist had the extra time, and the typist had nothing else to do. The cost is then just the out-of-pocket expense of supplies, the formalin, stains, alcohol, xylene, and other items needed; the glass slides, labels, and paper for the report. I have calculated this to be $5.08!

There is some justice, therefore, in the payments being made by local governments for the performance of medical-legal autopsies. As shown in the chapter on the medical-legal autopsy, many of the coroner's cases are done by hospital pathologists on a fee-for-service basis. The commonest payment to a hospital pathologist is about $200, with pathologists who have formal forensic training and certification receiving around $300. In addition, a fee of $25 to $50 is paid to the hospital where the autopsy is performed. Since the hospital has all the equipment in place and the personnel available, the payment seems quite reasonable, and it would be ridiculous to apply the $3,000 to $3,500 charge noted earlier as the real cost of the autopsy. Of course, the pathologist who ends up testifying in court as a result of a medical-legal autopsy should indeed be compensated additionally for his time and his expert opinion.

In geographic areas with well-organized departments of medical-legal investigation the pathologist is a salaried employee, and there are complete autopsy facilities for his work. It is difficult to assign a specific cost to a single autopsy, and the whole Institute of Legal Medicine where the work is done becomes a government expense. If this cost is divided by the number of autopsies, it is probably a great deal higher than the hospital autopsy. Another factor in the medical-legal autopsy which adds to the cost are the special studies which may be required, such as X-ray for location of bullets, toxicology studies for poisoning, special equipment for photographs and fingerprints, and the like.

Sometimes the pathologist is asked to perform an autopsy on the body of someone who is not either a medical-legal case, or a hospital death that would be his responsibility. There is no hospital chart to use for correlating the clinical findings with the results of the autopsy, so the usefulness of the autopsy as an educational procedure is indeed limited. It is appropriate in this situation for the pathologist to ask "Why this autopsy?" and alter his charges depending on the answer. It has always been my policy to perform such autopsies free of charge if the doctor who attended the deceased tells me that he would like the autopsy for his own scientific purposes. But if the autopsy is at the request of the survivors of the deceased, I have always felt justified in making a charge, particularly if the reason for the autopsy is the collection of insurance. I recall one case where an elderly patient with a long history of heart disease was found dead at the foot of a flight of stairs. The family physician, finding no bruises, was prepared to certify the death as due to a heart attack, but the family was anxious for an autopsy because if the death were due to a fall down the stairs, a double-indemnity clause in the deceased's insurance for death by accident would apply, and the family would be considerably enriched. I performed the autopsy and made a substantial charge, in spite of the fact that the autopsy showed clearly that the death was indeed due to a heart attack and there was no evidence to support a claim of a fall down the stairs. I'm sure that my autopsy was a great disappointment to the family, but I'm sure it saved them a long and expensive litigation which probably would not have succeeded in view of the opinion of the family doctor, had they decided to proceed with a suit without autopsy.

The insurance companies which reimburse hospitals generally decline to pay for autopsies as such, but they do recognize the autopsy service as a legitimate part of the general costs of operating a hospital; they recognize the inclusion of autopsy costs as part of the normal overhead. Occasionally an insurance company will want an autopsy, and will even offer to pay for it, but this is quite rare, and requires that the insurance company persuade the family to grant permission or the medical examiner to order the autopsy. It would occur only when some question directly affects the payment of a claim, and generally such questions arise within the purview of the insurance company long after the body has been buried or cremated. Obviously, if cremation has taken place, the question can never be answered, but occasionally bodies are exhumed for the purpose of autopsy at an insurance company's request and with family permission to answer some unresolved question.

Within the armed services of the United States, autopsies are performed routinely on bodies of individuals who have died in active service and the commander or the surgeon of the unit deems it necessary. As seen in chapter six, such autopsies do not require the permission of the family, and the costs are borne by the branch of the military service concerned.

Recently, the suggestion has been made that some costs might be saved by use of the problem-oriented autopsy. This is the performance of an autopsy directed at a specific problem; in other words, opening the body to study only the apparent disease which had been diagnosed by the clinical service. Thus, if the supposed cause of death as identified by the physicians who attended the patient in life is a heart attack, the pathologist will merely open the chest and examine the heart to confirm or deny the clinical diagnosis. There will be no check of the kidneys to see if blood-vessel narrowing might have caused high blood pressure, which in turn could have been at least a part of the cause of the heart attack. The congestion of the liver, with possible early damage to liver cells, will not be studied. And the examination of other organs for disease not related to the cause of death, but of very real significance to the family and to the science of medicine, will be skipped and the information lost on some possibility like early cancer of the lung, or a tiny but active nodule of the thyroid, or an ovarian cyst, or some other abnormality.

The problem-oriented autopsy is nothing new. It is the old, incomplete, cause-of-death autopsy which has been performed by lazy or overworked pathologists from the beginning of the science of pathology. It is probably better than no autopsy at all, but not much, since it gives a false picture of what is being done to investigate deaths. And the argument that there are substantial savings does not hold up, except for the costs of the pathologist's actual time, and in an adequately-staffed laboratory the pathologist should have time to contemplate, read, study, talk, and perform adequate autopsies.

In summary, it may be said that the autopsy is a complex procedure which, if charged at the same rate as other procedures in the hospital and the health care field, would be quite expensive, requiring as it does, highly trained personnel and complicated equipment. It is a testimony to the social necessity of autopsies that a method of paying the costs by spreading them over the whole area of health care and public support has evolved, making possible the availability of the autopsy with little worry about cost. The cost of supplies and other out-of-pocket items is minimal, so if the personnel and equipment are already available, the autopsy is a financial burden on no individual or segment of society. The social desirability of performing autopsies is therefore served, and society benefits.

CHAPTER SEVENTEEN

THE SOCIAL IMPORTANCE OF THE AUTOPSY

The previous chapters have discussed, either directly or by implication, a number of aspects of the autopsy procedure which clearly demonstrate its social importance. The need for autopsies in support of medical education for both the medical student and for the continuing education of practicing physicians is readily understandable, and the usefulness of careful investigation of unexplained or violent deaths to protect the public interest in matters of murder, suicide, and similar problems is equally clear. But there remain a number of other aspects of the autopsy procedure which contribute to the social usefulness, or better, the social necessity, of this activity.

Perhaps one aspect of autopsy that is of very great social importance is its use to avoid inappropriate guilt feelings among family members and others associated with the deceased. Certainly it is obvious that death of a loved one is surrounded with strong emotional reactions, and many people, faced with the fact of a death, wonder what they might have done to prevent it. This is especially traumatic when the death is at a younger age, or is very sudden and unexpected, and it is quite understandable that there can be strong feelings of guilt. Should the doctor have been called earlier? Should the patient's complaints been taken more seriously? Should Junior have been forced to shovel the snow, so Daddy wouldn't have done so, and had a heart attack?

Sometimes guilt is very real, and sometimes purely imaginary. Imaginary guilt is far more common.

Generally the determination of the exact cause of death demonstrates to the family and to the world that there was nothing that could have, or should have been done to alter the outcome of the disease that led to the death. Of course there are some very real exceptions. The athlete with the crushed vertebra in the neck probably would not have died if he had been moved more carefully after his injury, or the young woman with severe headache and loss of consciousness would probably have survived if she had been taken to the hospital instead of being put to bed to "sleep it off." While cases such as this are not very common, they do occur, and autopsies in these cases are very instructive; the finger of blame may indeed be pointed, but they serve to teach us all the appropriate measures to take in certain situations. But far more common is the relief the family is given by knowing that there was no way the death could have been prevented by any specific action they might have taken.

Perhaps the most telling example of the death-guilt for which autopsy is most therapeutic is the Sudden Infant Death Syndrome, called SIDS in many popular publications. The classic SIDS case is one in which an infant, generally less than a year old, is put to bed in apparent good health in the evening, and is found dead and cold in the morning, with no outcry or other indication of anything wrong during the night. This mysterious tragedy is all too often made even more tragic by the overwhelming destructive guilt feelings of the parents. Many happy marriages have been torn apart completely by the death of an infant and the self-blame or the blaming of one another by the father and mother of the child. It may be particularly traumatic if one parent or the other had punished the child shortly before the death.

It is only with autopsy that the parents can be reassured that nothing they might reasonably be expected to do would have altered the course in the particular case. The light spanking by Daddy the evening before had nothing to do with it. The medical-legal aspects of these problems was discussed in chapter nine, but here I want to emphasize the function of autopsy in the social problem of the relief of guilt. By being able to tell the bereaved couple that they could not have foreseen the event, and that they could not have prevented it, a great measure of natural guilt feelings can be relieved. And only by autopsy can the causes of preventable death be ruled out. In the case of true SIDS, the diagnosis can be made only by systematic exclusion of a number of specific anatomic diseases which might have caused the death. The true SIDS case is one in which pneumonia, cerebral hemorrhage, and other identifiable causes can be ruled out, and no true anatomic cause identified.

Every year, the development of new autopsy techniques, and the novel application of older procedures has reduced the number of truly unexplained sudden infant deaths. The identification of very subtle changes caused by virus pneumonia has moved many cases from the unexplained category. A pathologist friend of mine several years ago felt that he had identified a hemorrhage into the tissues around the spinal cord as a fairly consistent finding in these cases, and published an article in a medical journal about this finding, but other investigators have not supported this and feel that the apparent anatomic change is more likely an artifact caused by some variation in the technique of autopsy he used. The study goes on and on, but still there is a remainder of about fifty percent of the cases of sudden, unexplained and unexpected death of an apparently healthy, normal infant which may be classified as truly Sudden Infant Death Syndrome.

In most larger cities, the parents of infants who have died in this profoundly disturbing way have formed, often with professional encouragement by psychiatrists and social workers, support groups which have done a great deal to relieve guilt feelings, and to assist in prevention of further tragic destruction of personal relationships of the parents. Newly bereft parents are referred, generally by the family doctor or other professional person, to the group consisting of other parents who have been through a similar experience, and who have learned to cope with the tragedy. The process is much like any group therapy, like Alcoholics Anonymous, Reach to Recovery, and other similar organizations; the experienced members set themselves to helping the neophytes through their difficulties, and thereby get emotional help themselves. There is nothing more therapeutic in such situations than helping another person with a similar problem.

Through group therapy, professional advice and other mechanisms, guilt is dissipated and normal life permitted to resume. But one essential of the process in connection with SIDS is that an autopsy be done, so that an accurate determination of the cause of death — or lack of any anatomic cause — can be related to the parents. It is only through understanding the precise series of events that guilt can be laid down.

Sometimes autopsy is necessary to protect such parents, because all too often, parents are accused of child abuse resulting in death, when the actual cause is identifiable disease or SIDS. Only careful investigation can protect the distraught parents from vicious tongues and even legal accusations. Conversely, too, autopsy is important to reveal the cause of death if there has been actual child abuse. The situation then becomes murder, and should be treated as such. For this reason, as well as the protection of innocent parents, the medical-legal authorities routinely order autopsies to be done, under their authority to order autopsy, on any sudden or unexpected death. Using the same authority, medical school research groups, with the cooperation of local medical examiners, have conducted autopsies on SIDS infants in an effort to study the condition, in the hope of saving some lives through a better understanding of the problem.

Feeling guilt among friends and relatives is not restricted to infant deaths. Any death, no matter at what age it occurs, can have a profound emotional impact on the people involved. Guilt is a strong force operating in the human psyche, and it is likely to be found wherever illness and death are found. This points up the real reason for calling the doctor when illness occurs. The doctor is expected to relieve suffering and restore health to the best of his ability, but more importantly, the doctor is called to accept responsibility. The patient and his family need to feel that they have done the "right thing" if they are not to be plagued with doubt and guilt, and the "right thing" in the face of illness is to call the physician; the patient or his family can do no more, and the responsibility is shifted to the broad shoulders of the physician. Then, no matter what the outcome of the disease, cure, permanent disability, or death, there is not the burden of guilt over what might have been done differently.

The autopsy fits right into this pattern of relief of guilt by shifting responsibility. The family of the deceased has done the "right thing" by giving autopsy permission, and their responsibility to the deceased and to society generally, has been shifted away from where it can do its mischief. I recall vividly the death of a close friend of mine who was hospitalized following a heart attack and lung cancer, both related to his persistent use of cigarettes in spite of all urging from his family and friends, including me, to kick the habit. He died rather suddenly one morning in the intensive care unit of the hospital, and I urged the family to give permission for autopsy. It was granted, and I performed the procedure. In addition to confirmation of the healing heart attack and the early stages of lung cancer, I found the cause of death to be pulmonary embolism; a blood clot had formed in the leg veins due to his inactive, bedridden state in spite of all the standard treatments to prevent its formation, and it had broken loose and traveled through the veins and heart chambers to lodge in and completely block the arteries leading to the lungs. The family was greatly relieved when I was able to tell them that everything had been done properly, and that no one could have foreseen the event. Of course I didn't point out that he would not have been in the hospital bed at all if they had been able to get him to stop smoking years before, but they are intelligent, and I think they knew that anyway. Without the autopsy, they might have been plagued with doubts about the doctor, the hospital, the medications used, and their own role in the situation.

The autopsy can have further significance to the family of the deceased beyond the simple relief of guilt feelings. The exact cause of death is important to them and to society in many ways. Perhaps the most evident and compelling reason for autopsy is the discovery of previously unsuspected disease which may have great significance for other family members. Genetic disease may be revealed which has produced no symptoms in the deceased patient, but is of great importance to the survivors who are related to the patient. For instance, suppose a man in his middle age, driving on a dry, low-traffic highway, is seen to swerve suddenly off the road into a tree. His injuries do not explain the fact that he is clearly quite dead when he is pulled from the wreck. An autopsy reveals a heart attack; his coronary arteries are practically plugged with fatty deposits, and finally a diagnosis of familial hyperlipoproteinosis is made on further study. Such a diagnosis has great importance for the family members, who should be checked promptly for the same condition by simple laboratory tests. There is a great deal which can be done for any family member shown to have the same condition, if it is found early enough and treated promptly and adequately. The autopsy in such a case as this can save lives among members of the family of the deceased.

The presence of unsuspected contagious disease as a cause or at least a contributing cause of death is always a possibility which may be highly significant to family members and to the general public. It is regrettably familiar to encounter an attitude, even in the attending physician, of "We know why this patient died. Why do an autopsy?". But I have a pathologist's report in my files which gives a clear answer to this question. The report tells of the death of an old woman in a nursing home, who died apparently due to the familiar causes of arteriosclerotic heart disease and kidney failure. The intelligent family urged that autopsy be done in spite of the mild reluctance of the family doctor and the great inconvenience to everyone concerned, since nursing homes do not ordinarily have autopsy facilities. The autopsy revealed only mild heart and kidney disease, and the basic cause was active pulmonary tuberculosis. This was of great importance, as is readily realized, to not only the family members, but also to the personnel of the nursing home. Tuberculosis diagnosed in its early stages is readily treated, and several family members benefitted directly from the autopsy. The pathologist's report concludes, "I suspect that more frequent autopsies among older patients whose deaths are ascribed to well-defined chronic illnesses and occur at home or in extended care facilities, would reveal a higher incidence of tuberculosis than we now recognize."

Another example of the significance of the autopsy to the

family as well as to the general public is the discovery of unsuspected cancer in the body of the deceased. The cancer need not be the primary cause of death to be of great importance to family members, since it is known that there can be a very real tendency for certain cancers to run in particular families; someday indeed, a direct, clear, genetic transmission of at least some cancers may be demonstrated in certain family lines. A study at Cook County Hospital in Chicago in 1923 showed that cancers not suspected or incorrectly diagnosed by attending doctors occurred in 32.6% of the autopsies in a five-year period. A similar study was made at the Boston City Hospital forty-nine years later, and the percentage of incorrect diagnoses by clinicians who attended the patients in life was still about the same. These studies point out the fact that clinical diagnoses are often guesses — highly educated guesses, but guesses nevertheless, and autopsy is needed for the protection of the family and society generally, as well as for the accuracy of statistics on the causes of death, and for the education of doctors.

Many other examples of the advantages of the autopsy to family members can be given. Many genetic diseases are inherited in a recessive form, and when inherited from only one parent, there may be no evidence of clinical disease; it is only when both parents carry the trait or recessive form of the disease, that there is a likelihood of the clinical manifestation. Sex-linked recessive diseases are also familiar. One thinks of color blindness, where mothers with no apparent abnormality pass on the condition to half of their sons. Color blindness is obviously not a life-threatening disease. I've lived quite happily for many years with the condition, myself, but hemophilia, which is inherited in much the same pattern, is of great significance to anyone who might have inherited it. It is quite apparent that Queen Victoria passed hemophilia on to her daughters, who in turn produced hemophiliac sons in the Bourbon, Hapsburg, and Romanov families they married into. By luck — and the transmission of hemophilia is a lottery — the disease did not occur in Queen Victoria's own sons; the transmission is on the basis of a 50–50, flip-of-the-coin chance, so King Edward VII did not have the disease, nor any of his descendants. Obviously, autopsy is not essential for the diagnosis of hemophilia, nor can autopsy reveal the recessive trait in the mother, but many other inherited diseases can be proven by autopsy, and appropriate measures taken to either head off the disease in family members, or at least to suggest genetic counseling, where a couple contemplating marriage seeks advice, an effective and rewarding procedure.

The catalogue of genetic and familial diseases which require autopsy for their full definition and accurate diagnosis is quite long. To mention a few: there are the glycogen metabolism diseases: von Gierke's disease, Pompe's disease, Debrancher enzyme deficiency, and McArdle syndrome, all of which lead to the storage of glycogen (the starch-like food material which is one of the main forms of transmission and storage of energy in the body) in abnormal amounts in heart muscle, liver, skeletal muscles and elsewhere, and interferes with the vital functions of these and other organs. Familial hyperlipoproteinosis, with its buildup of cholesterol in the walls of arteries, has been noted earlier in this chapter. Brain diseases, such as Alzheimer's disease, Huntington's chorea and Friedreich's ataxia, require autopsy confirmation before the diagnosis can firmly be established. The list goes on and on. Suffice it to say, autopsy can be most important to the relatives of a patient dying of any one of a large number of hereditary diseases, and also to the relatives of a patient dying of nonhereditary causes, in whom hereditary disease is incidentally discovered at autopsy.

The importance of autopsy in the field of public health has already been suggested in the story of the old lady dying in the nursing home where autopsy revealed active tuberculosis as the primary cause of death. Tuberculosis, like syphilis, can be a real puzzler, because it can, depending on the organ affected, simulate so many other diseases. There is no way to be sure of any cause of death without autopsy, and the implications for the health of everyone who has had contact with the patient, often for years before the appearance of clinical disease, are of great significance should the actual cause be tuberculosis. This is what Public Health is all about: the protection of the public from transmissible disease, and the public in this case includes the family.

No doubt it is quite familiar to every reader that life

expectancy has been greatly expanded in the current century. To avoid argument, I won't quote any statistics on this, since various calculations have been made and they don't always agree precisely, but everyone agrees that the chances of surviving to an older age have been vastly improved in recent years. It is clear that medical knowledge is primarily responsible for this increase in longevity. Many people think in terms of the doctor at the bedside treating sick individuals more successfully, because of better knowledge and better medication, and this is partially true; we have drugs like penicillin, but the greatest increase in life expectancy is directly a consequence of public health measures. The doctor at the bedside may save individual lives, but the public health physician saves the lives of whole populations. The apparent elimination of smallpox, the tremendous reduction in the incidence of measles, and the virtual disappearance of diphtheria are a few examples of how populations rather than individuals have been protected from diseases that, over the years, have led to so many premature deaths. And so many of the public health advances would never have been possible without the background information from autopsies of persons affected by these diseases. Autopsy is required to identify specifically and directly the nature of a particular disease which constitutes a hazard for the general public.

Another aspect of public health work in lengthening the human life span is found in the systematic work following up drug misadventures, and preventing unwise applications of newly discovered medications. The Food and Drug Administration (FDA) has been criticized severely for withholding licenses on new drugs which might save lives, but this criticism has rarely been justified. Most of the FDA's work has been a very valuable protection to the citizens of our country. One has only to think of the thalidomide tragedy, where large numbers of children were born without arms, legs, or both as a result of pregnant women using the tranquilizer during their first three months of pregnancy. We should be very grateful for the reluctance of the FDA's refusal to release the drug before it had been thoroughly tested. The abnormality caused by thalidomide was painfully clear without autopsy as far as the arms and legs were concerned, but autopsy was and is necessary to discover the internal abnormalities which accompanied the absence of arms and legs; nearly every external abnormality of this type is accompanied by internal congenital diseases and abnormal structures.

The proliferation of new medicines and novel surgical procedures makes the performance of autopsy essential if the public is to be protected from dangerous manipulations while it is given the advantages of new discoveries. Animal studies are regarded as most important in the studies of safety and effectiveness before new medicines are released for human use, but it must be remembered that each animal species is different in many subtle ways, and reactions of animals to drugs may not always operate as reliable predictors of reactions in humans. As a result, human reactions must be studied and recorded to complete the picture after animal trials have indicated the probable safety and effectiveness of the material or procedure. New surgical operations, and other modes of therapy such as radiation, ultrasound, and other physical procedures, must be checked for their ultimate effect in human beings with the same thoroughness as drug therapy. Autopsy is practically the only way to do this with the sort of completeness that is necessary; especially valuable is the autopsy of a case which has died of some cause unrelated to the experimental treatment. If a patient with a new, experimental heart valve prosthesis which has been working perfectly, for instance, is killed in an auto accident, the autopsy is most urgently needed to document the success of the new device. Diagnostic procedures, too, need to be checked for possible damage to the individual as well as new therapeutic techniques.

My own contact with the experimental drug problem occurred while I was in residency training. A twelve-year-old boy with a history of epilepsy had been treated with a new experimental drug under careful, university-sponsored supervision, but he suddenly developed profound jaundice and died. I had the responsibility of speaking to the family to get autopsy permission, and in spite of my most persuasive arguments the family flatly refused to sign the permission. It was the one of the greatest disappointments of my medical career; if I could have obtained the permission, the autopsy would surely have shown the nature of the liver damage which resulted in the jaundice, and possibly shown a way that such damage could be prevented while continuing the use of the medication. As it was, the medicine had to be withdrawn and never used again, and the loss to medical knowledge is incalculable. I still feel the pain of this defeat, many years later, and reflect on how many lives might have been changed and made more bearable if I had been able to persuade the parents to grant autopsy permission.

Another aspect of autopsy in relation to the family and its interests should be mentioned, although it can be used only rarely to persuade a family to grant permission because it can backfire. Many insurance policies exclude payment for deaths resulting from certain diseases or certain causes of death. The exclusion of payment for suicide within two years of the inception of the policy is perhaps the most familiar of these excluded causes. Sometimes causes of death such as tuberculosis or other diseases that are accepted to be a government responsibility (in that public facilities are provided for caring for people with these diseases) are specifically excluded. If an excluded disease or cause of death is highly suspected, then the family may grant permission in hopes that some other cause will be found and the insurance claim paid. But all too often, from the family's point of view, the autopsy will confirm the cause and the family will lose the insurance, and lose the opportunity of even suggesting that the cause could have been otherwise and they therefore should be paid. Such an autopsy does, however, protect the public from unjustified claims and increased costs of insurance to all. I remember a case where I traveled a considerable distance to perform an autopsy in a funeral home, having been called by the family after the medical examiner declined to order an autopsy and ruled the case a suicide. I performed the examination, which clearly confirmed the suicide diagnosis, and the family lost the insurance claim. I was never paid for that autopsy.

Many insurance policies carry a double-indemnity clause, which applies in case the death was caused by accident. Personally, I have never understood the rationale for such a clause, because the purpose of insurance should be to provide for financial needs of the survivors, and their needs should be covered by a specific amount of insurance. I fail to see how their needs would be twice as great if the death was caused by accident. Indeed, it is likely to be less, because the death would probably be quicker and not attended by the costs of long hospitalization. The higher premium for double-indemnity payment for death under certain circumstances seems foolish and wasteful, but these clauses are very common, and often an autopsy is needed to support claims made. Conversely, sometimes an autopsy will reveal that an apparent accident was actually nonaccidental, and the family may lose money that they might otherwise have collected. Again I can cite, however, the value of protection of the public from unjustified claims. Exact knowledge has tremendous value in relation to the collection of insurance proceeds, just as it has in so many other fields that are important to society.

A pathologist in New York tells of an interesting case: an older man with a known history of heart disease and previous heart attacks was recovering from an operation for aortic aneurysm, a leaking major blood vessel which threatened to burst. He was going to bed, and stumbled against the bedside table, collapsed and died. His widow was much opposed to autopsy, but the surgeon who was understandably anxious to know if a failure of his operation or a new heart attack had caused the death, finally persuaded her to sign a permission. The pathologist found that neither of the suspected diagnoses was the cause, but that the patient had died from a ruptured spleen, injured when he stumbled against the bedside table, an accident which could have happened to anyone, and which was not related to the operation, the heart disease, or any other suspected cause. The widow consequently received a great deal of unexpected money because his accident insurance had a double-indemnity policy for accidental death. Without autopsy, the case would surely have been certified as a heart attack, the widow would never have been paid double, and the surgeon would always have wondered if the actual cause was a failure of his operation.

Medical research is another field in which the social importance of the autopsy is amply demonstrated. The tremendous strides that have been made in understanding the reactions of the immune system, both the normal protective reactions and the abnormal reactions which produce disease states, have depended on autopsy, along with animal studies and test-tube experiments; without autopsy, these advances could never have been made. This is only one example of the many fields of medical research which have been pushed forward in recent years. In chapter eight, I have spoken of the recent development of the electron microscope as a tool of diagnosis; the autopsy procedure enables the investigator to take a fresh look, with the electron beam, at the disease states which were previously studied with the light-microscope. This has resulted in many startling and innovative concepts regarding the nature of some diseases that were previously poorly understood. There is so much to learn about the human body, and the autopsy provides material by which this learning can take place.

We have already spoken of the function of the autopsy in connection with organ donation, the spare-parts procedure whereby kidneys, hearts, and other organs have been replaced and dying patients given a new life, often lasting for many years. It would be very hard to argue that autopsy was not socially useful in such cases. There is no need to belabor this point further; it speaks for itself.

A newly developing field of pathology related to public health work is that of environmental pathology. This is the study of disease as it is related to the world around the patient, and its dependance on the autopsy procedure is very important. Certain of the diseases studied, such as the effects of sunlight in producing skin cancer — a most important and sadly neglected problem — can be followed successfully by biopsy techniques, and autopsy is not essential. But other problems, such as the production of unusual tumors of the lung and associated tissues by exposure to asbestos, could never have been attacked with any hope of success without the use of autopsies. All sorts of industrial solvents, dusts, and other environmental factors would never have been understood as disease producers — even to the limited extent they are understood today — without repeated autopsies of their victims. The conditions which result from exposure to excessive heat and excessive cold could never have been demonstrated, and measures could not have been devised to treat and protect those affected, without the autopsies conducted on those who died of heat or cold. Sudden changes in pressure, such as blast injury, explosive decompression and related conditions, have required autopsy for understanding and there is still a long way to go in fully understanding these conditions. We need autopsy, autopsy, and autopsy to make any progress in trying to protect the individual and the general public from all sorts of disease-causing conditions, both in industry, and in the nonindustrial (even recreational) environment.

Sports medicine, another developing field of medical care, likewise owes a great debt to autopsies performed on those who have died on the playing fields, the ski trails, and elsewhere, in their search for personal satisfaction or in their effort to entertain others. There is no area in health care that does not depend in part, and sometimes almost in whole, on the autopsies performed on the bodies of those who have left us.

The remaining area of social importance of the autopsy is the law. I have discussed this to some extent in chapter eight from the point of view of the medical examiner and his work, but I should not leave the subject of social importance without pointing out again the absolute, compelling necessity for autopsies in both civil and criminal cases before the law. Of course, homicide is the most dramatic aspect of this, and very few detective stories revolve around anything else but homicide. Indeed, I think of only one classic detective story which didn't center on murder, Edgar Allen Poe's tale, *The Gold Bug*. Homicide investigation is rarely complete or definitive without autopsy, whether in fiction or in real life. I doubt that anyone would argue that murder investigation is not of social importance, but there are many other legal questions not involving murder where autopsy is urgently needed to establish facts and permit the administration of real justice. Workmen's compensation, for instance, is profoundly affected by autopsy, and environmental pathology, which I have just discussed, have tremendous legal implications. The investigation of deaths by accident is essential to reveal hazards for which legal actions can provide remedies, and the legal implications of insurance have already been discussed. Suffice it to say, there is rarely a case involving the death that results in court action that does not require an autopsy for real justice to be done.

In summary, there is rarely any valid reason not to perform an autopsy on the body of any deceased person, whether the death occurs in a hospital or at home, in the factory or far afield. The results of the autopsy are needed for the information and the protection of the health of surviving family members, and for the advancement of medical education and research. The protection of the public from communicable diseases, environmental hazards, and criminal activity is dependant in case after case upon the precise determination of the cause of death. There is no apparent objection to the performance of the autopsy beyond the primitive anti-intellectualism which is regrettably all too common. No basic religious concept forbids it, and every human value encourages it. There is no loss except the time and materials needed to complete the study, and the hazard to the pathologist and his assistants is minimal and insignificant if properly managed. All in all, there is no reason not to do autopsies on every death, and there is every reason to do so.

I like to recall the motto which one famous pathologist had emblazoned above his working area: *Here the Dead Delight to Serve the Living.*